PRAISE FOR *PARENTIN* *~~~~ ~~~~~~~~~*

This book, co-authored by one of our leading geriatricians, offers a unique and sometimes moving blend of information, insight, compassion, advocacy, and humour. It should be a valuable resource for families needing to help frail parents who have many things wrong at once, but who must deal with health care systems that largely prefer people to get sick with one illness at a time.

Kenneth Rockwood, MD, FRCPC
Professor of Geriatric Medicine, Dalhousie University
Past President, the Canadian Society of Geriatric Medicine

From my professional experiences I know that what people need is practical and understandable information. That is exactly what *Parenting Your Parents* is, and for me personally it has been invaluable in helping me to support my aging relatives. My hope is that my own children read it one day so I too can be the beneficiary of the advice.

Nancy Webb
Vice-President, Public Affairs
Baycrest Centre for Geriatric Care

As a minister I come into contact with hundreds of people who are facing the struggles that Bart Mindszenthy and Michael Gordon speak about in *Parenting Your Parents*. I also faced these same issues with my own parents before they passed away. I have to say that the authors give not only timely advice, but practical, useful advice that can easily be understood and immediately applied. I should know; I used their advice with my own parents and have offered it to others in my capacity as minister of a large city church and counselling practice.

Dr. Rev. John Niles

Michael Gordon has combined his extensive experience as a physician caring for elderly patients with his warmth and humanity to create, along with his co-author Bart Mindszenthy, a unique book that will be a source of information, advice, and great comfort for anyone involved in the care of an aging parent.

Eliot A. Phillipson, MD
Sir John and Lady Eaton Professor of Medicine Emeritus
Past Chair, Department of Medicine, University of Toronto

I have recommended *Parenting Your Parents* to many of my faculty colleagues who are facing the challenge of caring for their aging parents. This book, which discusses these challenges eloquently, is a very valuable resource. The last person who borrowed my copy must have agreed, because he never returned it!

Anne Sclater, MD, FRCPC
Professor and Chair of Medicine, Memorial University of Newfoundland

The personal stories of other families encountering the same obstacles I faced acted as a lightning rod to recharge my batteries to enable me to do what I knew I had to do as the only provider for my aging parents. It is quite evident that the introduction was written by a man who had a great love for his own parents; I had the minister read several paragraphs from it at my mother's funeral service.

Bruce West

As my widowed mother-in-law slowly descends into dementia, *Parenting Your Parents* has helped me and my partner find support and direction as we pick our way through a minefield of grief, stress, and frantic concern.

Kathee Muzin

Bart Mindszenthy was the keynote speaker at a Prime Plus™ course I attended last year. I was so impressed with his candid insight to eldercare that I immediately read his book *Parenting Your Parents*. Not only do I recommend this book to all my clients facing eldercare, but the philosophy and advice found in *Parenting Your Parents* is the foundation of our eldercare practice.

Lawrence Zinman, BComm, CA, CFE
Partner, Schwartz Levitksy Feldman LLP, Chartered Accountants

I often recommend *Parenting Your Parents* to my clients. The senior executives in large corporations are increasingly having to juggle demanding careers and the care of elderly parents. This book gives them a great resource while allowing them to connect with others in the same situation.

Hélène Beauchemin
Executive Coach

Parenting Your Parents is not only an excellent resource, but it is a book that provides a level of comfort. The case studies sensitively and realistically tell stories that validated my feelings and concerns during a difficult time. Although every person's situation and relationship with their aging parents is unique there are many messages for everyone in *Parenting Your Parents*.

Anne Yeager

As the only child of an only child, I see the story of my family in the pages of this book — it's comforting, illuminating, and a great resource all in one!

Cindy LaValley

This book was a survival handbook in dealing with my aging parents. Reading it made me realize that the difficulties my siblings and I are experiencing with our parents are not unique. The stories are sad, funny, and honest, and the guidelines are practical.

Lawrie Senders

PARENTING YOUR PARENTS

Support Strategies for Meeting the Challenge of Aging in the Family

BART MINDSZENTHY AND MICHAEL GORDON, MD

THE DUNDURN GROUP
TORONTO

Copy-Editor: Jennifer Bergeron
Design: Andrew Roberts
Printer: Webcom

Library and Archives Canada Cataloguing in Publication

Mindszenthy, Bart J., 1946-
    Parenting your parents : support strategies for meeting the
challenge of
aging in the family / Bart Mindszenthy and Michael Gordon. -- 2nd ed., rev.
and expanded

ISBN 1-55002-552-X

    1. Aging parents--Care. 2. Parent and adult child. I. Gordon,
Michael, 1941-
II. Title.

HQ1063.6.M55 2005   306.874   C2005-900176-3

1   2   3   4   5   09 08   07   06   05

  Canada

ONTARIO ARTS COUNCIL
CONSEIL DES ARTS DE L'ONTARIO

Conseil des Arts du Canada
Canada Council for the Arts

We acknowledge the support of the Canada Council for the Arts and the Ontario Arts Council for our publishing program. We also acknowledge the financial support of the Government of Canada through the Book Publishing Industry Development Program and The Association for the Export of Canadian Books, and the Government of Ontario through the Ontario Book Publishers Tax Credit program, and the Ontario Media Development Corporation's Ontario Book Initiative.

Care has been taken to trace the ownership of copyright material used in this book. The author and the publisher welcome any information enabling them to rectify any references or credit in subsequent editions.

J. Kirk Howard, President

Printed and bound in Canada.
Printed on recycled paper.

www.dundurn.com

Dundurn Press
8 Market Street, Suite 200
Toronto, Ontario, Canada
M5E 1M6

Gazelle Book Services Limited
White Cross Mills
Hightown, Lancaster, England
LA1 4X5

Dundurn Press
2250 Military Road
Tonawanda NY
U.S.A. 14150

To our parents,
whose lifelong legacy of love and caring
serves to guide and inspire us.

TABLE OF CONTENTS

Acknowledgements 9

Foreword *by Sandie Rinaldo* 11

Introduction: The Case for the Cause: Parent Care *Is* a Major
Social Issue and Challenge 13

Parenting Your Parents: Stepping into the Unknown 17

The Rocky Road of Responsibility 26

NINETEEN FAMILY CASE STUDIES

Control: Laying on the Guilt Trip 33

Surgery: Weighing the Odds 40

Eldertravel: Balancing Risks and Benefits 48

Independence: Helping Parents Live Their Lives 55

Breaking the Mold: The Rebellious Grandmother 63

Culture Clash: Pitting Values against Needs 70

Substance Abuse: Drinking All Day Keeps Reality Away 78

Sexuality, Romance, and the Family: When Children Worry
about Their Parents 85

Tapping the Human Spirit: It's Never Too Late to Create 92

Siblings: In Charge and On the Attack 99

The Conflicted Single Child: A Confusing Battle of Priorities 106

The Stroke: Sudden Challenges and Changes 115

Dementia and Depression: Reading the Signs 121

Advancing Dementia: When Life Gets More Difficult 129

We're On Our Own: How to Plan for the Future 137

Finding a New Life: Corrections and Concerns 144

Decision Time: Planning for the Inevitable   151
End of Life: Caring and Sharing   157
Moving On: Living Life without a Loved One   164

Our Own Experiences

Roz and Max
by Michael Gordon   172
A Week of Trauma Sets the Stage for Hurt and Hope
by Bart Mindszenthy   201

Tools to Help You

Personal Parenting Planner   240
A Financial Primer: Managing Your Parents' Finances   275
Resource Directory   282

ACKNOWLEDGEMENTS

A special thank you to those who gave us encouragement and support most every day throughout the process of writing this book initially, and while revising it for this second edition: Michael's wife, Gilda Berger, and sister, Diane Gordon; Bart's partner, Gail Roberts, his ever-inquiring and interested father, and his persistent daughter, Andrea, and son-in-law and freshly minted physician, Julian.

A warm thank you to Dr. Robert Horvath, who arranged for us to meet and discover that, indeed, we could work very well together.

Special appreciation to Sandra DeAthe for her detailed, dogged, and dedicated work in helping to revise and update the Resource Directory, which is such a valuable tool. Her intense research and most welcomed contribution has made this new edition all the more useful. The original directory was based on many listings provided for the first edition of this book by Caroline Tapp-McDougall, publisher of *Solutions* magazine, and the Baycrest Centre for Geriatric Care. Others who assisted with the original directory were Glenn Hildebrand in Winnipeg, Manitoba; Gerard Godbout in Hull, Quebec; Rod Stanely in Summerside, P.E.I.; Leanne Tait in Yellowknife, Northwest Territories; Joel Weiner, the former Regional Director for Ontario for Health Canada, and his staff; and all the nice people in provincial ministries and with various associations who were so kind with their time.

The revised and expanded Personal Parenting Planner is now more complete thanks to the insights and input of David Wm. Brown, CFP, CLU, ChFC, RHU, partner at the independent financial and estate planning firm of Al G. Brown & Associates. We also welcomed barrister and solicitor Allan Strader's review of the planner.

Thanks, too, to John Wright and Ipsos-Reid for providing research data on the issue of parent and eldercare.

Also many thanks to Mona Munro and Renne Climens of the Department of Social Work at the Baycrest Centre for Geriatric Care and Irma Baumlisberger for their input and comments.

Finally, we are delighted with Dundurn Press's keen interest in this book, starting with Tony Hawke, who expressed a deep conviction that the time was right and ripe for *Parenting Your Parents*, and Beth Bruder, who made the original connection because she knew first-hand of the need. Thanks also to Barry Jowett, our superb editorial coordinator, who did a magnificent job keeping us on track, and the staff who worked on the production of the book: Jennifer Bergeron, Andrew Roberts, and Jennifer Scott.

And, to all of you who were willing to tell us the stories of your own experiences ... thank you for sharing openly your personal and family challenges.

FOREWORD

by Sandie Rinaldo

Who can help but learn from Boris, Bob, Ivan, and Sophie? Ivan and Sophie are elderly parents who've been encouraged by their well-intentioned sons, Boris and Bob, to leave their home in Red Deer and move to Montreal to be near them. What begins as a tender reunion quickly sours as family pressures intermingle with filial responsibilities. Wives are unhappy. Grandchildren disinterested. And, sadly, Ivan and Sophie feel misplaced and long to return to their old way of life.

Theirs is but one of nineteen anecdotes the authors have collected in this storytelling anthology that explores an important and timely topic.

You might recognize yourself in Boris and Bob; or in Sylvia, who must find the resources to care for her mother, Lee Ann, while she recovers from surgery; or Edna Delaney's four children, whose sibling rivalry and mutual mistrust have caused Edna enormous stress; or Dorothy Miller, whose family must cope with her advancing dementia.

From surviving a stroke to reining in a rebellious grandmother, from angst to xenophobia, the authors let the case studies carry the book. They chart the challenges through the stories of families who have encountered a myriad of personal and family trials and tribulations, and offer sound, logical advice based on years of personal and professional experience. Perhaps that's what makes this book unique. It's not a sophisticated treatise laced with medical lingo, but rather the kind of read that's reminiscent of descriptive fiction. And yet, the stories and characters in *Parenting Your Parents* are real.

Two real gems round out the book: the Personal Parenting Planner, which serves as a status check, a fact-gathering repository, and an action planner, and the Resource Directory — a who-to-call lifeline. Both have been updated and revised for this second edition of the book.

As the sandwich generation, we live in a new reality, where isolation is a factor, and where families and neighbourhood roles are changing. We have much to learn from the shared experiences of others.

Boris and Bob taught me that sometimes it's wiser to help parents live their lives their way instead of pushing an agenda because you think it might be better for them. My dad will thank them for my newfound wisdom. He thrives on independence, and as long as he is healthy and of good mind, he should continue to live life to the fullest.

Consider this book a valuable resource.

Sandie Rinaldo
January 2005

THE CASE FOR THE CAUSE:

Parent Care Is a Major Social Issue and Challenge

W elcome to the revised edition of *Parenting Your Parents*. This edition includes a number of new case studies, a new resource tool to help you better understand the considerations for managing your parents' finances, an expanded Personal Parenting Planner that includes key financial considerations as well as an opportunity to score your parents' current level of vulnerability, and a completely updated Resource Directory. We also bring you up to date on our own personal experiences.

Why? Because caring for our aging parents and other elderly loved ones is now a major familial and societal issue in Canada, across North America, and around the world.

The numbers speak for themselves. And the numbers are awesome. For example, The Empire Club of Canada asked Ipsos-Reid, the national polling and research firm, to conduct a national survey in mid-September 2004 about what the major issues Canadians believe they will have to confront a decade from now. A substantial majority — 72 percent — identified "services for the elderly and their specific home and healthcare needs" as the number one issue that the federal and provincial governments will have to face.

According to the 2003 figures from Statistics Canada, there are nearly 5. 5 million Canadians sixty years of age and older. Some are doing remarkably well for their age, some are in line with statistical expectations, and many are in failing health — physically or mentally or both. They all need, and most expect, our care and concern.

As they become more frail, our elderly parents and other loved ones will require more of our time and patience and commitment to ensure they'll live their closing years in as much comfort, dignity, and safety as possible.

In fact, physicians acknowledge that eldercare is extremely demanding on their professional time and on the health care system in general. They point out that the elderly, especially those over eighty, usually require more time for an appointment because they tend to have more complex medical issues that must be addressed. Frequently, family members visit the doctor with their parent to assist, and that, too, requires extra time for explanations. As well, the elderly generally have doctors' appointments more often than healthier young or middle-aged persons. Plus, if hospitalized, elderly patients more often need a higher level of care and treatment and longer periods for recovery.

Statistics Canada projects that by 2011, there'll be more than 7 million Canadians sixty years of age or older.

Presently, more than 9.25 million Canadians are between the ages of forty and fifty-nine, and the majority of them have living parents and in-laws who increasingly will need their help and support in some way. A 2002 Statistics Canada report indicated that more than 4 million Canadians aged forty-five to seventy-five and older were providing informal care to those sixty-five and older who were experiencing long-term health problems.

The same study showed that hundreds of thousands of Canadian women and men are experiencing serious workplace consequences as a result of providing what is termed "informal" parent and eldercare. They've reported impacts ranging from reduced hours of work to lost income; from turning down job opportunities to actually quitting work. The study also demonstrates that there are very real and tangible negative consequences for their social activities, holiday plans, actual expenses, and even sleep patterns and personal health.

So the implications are clear and imperative to address, as the baby boomers age and become the next and greatest wave to challenge the health care system and the family structure.

There is more data to drive home the range and scope of the issue. Ipsos-Reid notes that 73 percent of adult Canadians have living parents or in-laws. About 24 percent of this adult population believes that at some point they'll have to help their parents.

Another recent Ipsos-Reid study found that 25 percent of Canadian adults acknowledge that Alzheimer's disease has already been diagnosed for someone in their family circle.

In a survey conducted among employees with benefit plans (some 71 percent of the Canadian workforce), Ipsos-Reid identified that 32 percent are responsible for eldercare, while 12 percent are responsible for caring for both children under the age of eighteen and an elderly family member. The survey also revealed that one-third of the workers who care for elderly family members average twenty-three hours of caregiving per month, and 17 percent indicate they'll have to take more time off in the next two years for those responsibilities.

Yet another study by the firm found that 17 percent of Canadian adults currently have either parents or in-laws living with them or expect that one or both parents will live with them as they get older.

Finally, as a personal favour to the authors, Ipsos-Reid polled a representative sampling of Canadians and found two truly significant gaps that we believe are imperative to recognize and deal with throughout the process of caring for our aging parents. The first is that only 36 percent of adult Canadians have discussed candidly with their parents or in-laws long-term care plans so that they'll understand their expectations for assistance and care as they age. The second is that 63 percent of Canadians say they'll feel guilty unless they can adequately provide their parents or in-laws with the kind of help or social assistance they'll need at some point.

The fact remains, as research shows, that we're generally opting to avoid the very critical discussions we should have while our parents are well because those kinds of discussions are uncomfortable and usually downright difficult. However, those are precisely the kinds of discussions we must have if we're to do the right things, the right way, at the right time.

As for guilt: it comes with the territory. We'll latch onto guilt unless we plan, talk, build bridges with our parents and family in a timely way, and do the best we can.

To exacerbate the challenges facing us, recently released data from the 2002 General Social Survey by the Canadian government found that there were more than seven hundred thousand Canadians aged forty-five to sixty-four who had unmarried children under the age of twenty-five living at home, and also aging parents to support. Surely this demonstrates that what we often call the "sandwich generation" has stresses and strains that will exact a toll of some kind, in some way.

All this underscores the point that caring for our aging parents is a major personal and social issue. There isn't any shortcut. There aren't any easy answers.

Yet, given our social structure, there should be more government recognition for what we do in the home for our parents, which actually relieves the pressure on the health care system.

So welcome to the wonderful new world of parenting your parents.

It's a world of tingling emotions and stress and fear and, very often, of finding new bonds and levels of love and affection. It's a journey of discovering conflicting personal weaknesses and strengths. It's all about recognizing that we are extensions of our parents, whether we like it or not, and understanding that the needs they have as they age and decline are heartfelt weights we must carry.

It's a new, uncharted path in the process of discovering how human we really are.

Bart Mindszenthy and Michael Gordon
January 2005, Toronto

PARENTING YOUR PARENTS

Stepping into the Unknown

They're now very old and frail, my parents. I'm told by so many that I'm fortunate to still have them. The people who tell me this lost their own parents when they were still relatively young — in their late sixties and early seventies.

As we start to work on this book, my mother is eighty-six years old, and my father is getting close to ninety-six. They're fragile. They're proud. They're fiercely determined. They're more the exception than the rule, given their ages.

They still live in their North York home, and every day they get up, wash, dress, make their beds, and eat their breakfast. They work very hard at making their lives as normal as they can, and it's somewhat like watching a movie in slow motion for most of us, since they just move more slowly and everything takes longer.

I'm proud of them. I'm afraid for them. I'm confused about my role, my obligation. I know we're marking time. I can see it every time I'm with them. Their strength and determination are fading and being replaced by sheer will and a kind of day-to-day disciplined routine that keeps them going.

They're very social, but also very private. They don't want people they don't know to come and help them. It's almost like some kind of threat. So they depend on me — and on a young married woman who comes three or four times a week to help them bathe, clean, cook, and run errands. I really don't know what I'd do without her help, how I'd cope with where we are in the end game of their lives.

And that's precisely where we are. The end game. They know it. I know it. We don't talk about it too much, but that's the reality we elect to ignore as often and for as long as we can.

My parents are unique and amazing. But so are all parents. There are no two sets alike, anywhere, ever. They're what we get at birth. They're the link to the past and our passports to the future. Most parents do the best they can, no matter what we think or feel in the course of life. They weren't "trained" in parenthood, so they made up rules and procedures as they went along. Or they read Dr. Spock and followed his strict guidelines, which have long since been denounced.

No matter which course they took, our parents struggled and strove to do what they thought was best for us in preparing us for the future. They imparted to us lifelong values and beliefs, often without our realizing it, that we, perhaps, too seldom challenge, but rather uphold without always understanding them. Our parents were, and often still are, more influential in our lives than we can ever acknowledge or even comprehend.

Parents are special. We love to love them, and we sometimes try to hate them. There are times we see them as an intrusive burden and long to cut the chains that bind us. But seldom, if ever, can we walk away from them. Or even want to.

Our parents are simply there — with us, for us. They are an integral part of our world — in our minds, in our lives, sometimes in the way. Never out of the way, until they die. And when they do, there is an immense emotional outflow of fear, love, loss, anger, and confusion. For these are the people who so influenced who and what we are today, and, more often than not, we don't even realize the impact they've had until they're gone.

We who wrote this book, and everyone reading it, are trapped by the indisputable fact that the old rules and structures that drove the family compact are virtually non-existent. Just consider: Our parents, most of whom were born in the first third of the twentieth century, were reared with values and family and social expectations that have radically changed in the past forty years. The difference between their paradigm and ours is probably greater than that of any other back-to-back generations.

Advances in medicine and major improvements in our quality of life mean people are living longer than ever — and our parents are the first generation to truly benefit — but not without paying a price.

We baby boomers and our children are more mobile than any generation before. We change where we live and work more often than ever. For many, that means there is the added dimension of distance between our parents and us.

The two-income family is commonplace, putting added pressure on us to spend time helping our own children, who are more often returning to the family nest at some point in their lives for a period of time. So there is less time to spend supporting parents in need than there was in the 1950s and 1960s, when the wife and mother of a family had a traditional role as homemaker and supporter that was clear and socially acceptable at the time.

There is a relatively new phenomenon of "multi-parent children": those whose parents have divorced and remarried or are living in common-law relationships. New challenges centre around emotions, loyalties, and priorities in considering how best to apply attention and energy in supporting not two, but possibly three or four "parents."

The major changes that governments have introduced in the past decade to cut costs and taxes have resulted in a strain on services for the aging offered by the not-for-profit sector.

Where does all this leave you and me? Usually, between a rock and a hard place that is stifling, intimidating, and frightening.

But all of us who have aging parents want to help them. The challenge is to help them without becoming captives in the process: captives to parent care and parent over-dependency. It's a tough balancing act, with no set rules and myriad but confusing support mechanisms. We're in uncharted waters, and the water is deep and cold and treacherous.

So back to my parents and how I came to know them.

Late on the evening of June 12, 1946, a midwife nudged and eased me from my mother's warm, safe womb into the confusing, devastated, hurtful, hateful, hungry world of post-World War II Europe.

And so I was born, the only child of my parents. Hungarian by birth, but a citizen of a new world. For the first few years of my life, we lived from hand to mouth as refugees in Bavaria. We were "DPs" — displaced persons: people who had lost their homeland, their homes, and all their possessions. People who were trying to find a new life because the war had taken everything from them. Then, in the summer of 1949, we were sponsored to come to America, the land of dreams and hope.

We arrived in Detroit with one suitcase. My father weighed all of ninety-nine pounds, and my mother was ill. But we managed to cross the Atlantic on an old, eleven-thousand-ton troop carrier crammed with others seeking a new life in a new world.

There was nothing glamorous about my early years. My parents worked hard at learning English and at their jobs, and they tried as best they could to give me all that a little kid might expect. Except in my case, for the first number of years, what I got was used clothing and hand-me-down toys.

I remember a lot of things that aren't terribly relevant. What is relevant is that they tried so hard to bring joy and direction to my world, and they gave it with as much love and affection as they knew how.

Now, more than half a century later, we're into role reversal. I am the "parent," and they are the ones who need care, attention, support, and loving. But now we're in another country — Canada, where I came in 1969, and where my parents followed after retirement in 1973.

My father is now legally blind; his bodily functions are working relatively well, considering his age, but everything in his day-to-day world is happening in slow motion. My mother's memory is faltering, mainly because of the sleeping pills to which she's become addicted.

I live twelve kilometres away from them — not a big distance except during rush hours and snowstorms. I make it a point to see them every other day, to spend some time talking with them and doing things for them.

As I look back on where we've been and where we are, what I sense and feel is that through all the turmoil and upheaval of the past five-plus decades, my parents did the best they could to protect and help me, to make my little world safe and secure. And as I listen and learn from others, I hear that they, too, for the most part, remember parents who did the best they could to protect and help them, wherever they were at the time. And that's maybe the single most important thing we all have in common: parents who did the best they could for us.

Now, we've got to return the favour. We've got to help them as they become more and more helpless, just like they helped us when we were helpless. Nice and noble to say, but in today's world, it's very hard to do. If we're honest with ourselves, we know that while we love our parents, becoming their caregivers is not something we want to do. And we're unsure, because most of us don't quite know how to approach the task in the best way possible.

So the bottom line question is this: Do we have the will, the energy, the power, the resources, and the commitment to do it? Or, put another way, do we have a moral choice? Yes, we're ever thoughtful of our careers. Yes, we want to be secure financially. Yes, we want our kids to forge their own lives while we help them the best we can. And yes, we live in a confusing, uncertain, ever-changing world. But aside from all that, we have parents who are aging and in various conditions of decay (because what else can we call it if we're facing the cold facts?) and fully cognizant that we're all marking time.

So here we are, in our forties and fifties — and even into our sixties — with a growing set of unwanted responsibilities that we can either address or ignore. And it all comes down to choices. Hard choices. Confusing and challenging choices. And that's what this book is all about.

Whether or not we agree with what our parents did in the past or what they're doing now, they are our parents. Were it not for them, we wouldn't be. But we are. And because we are, we must care for them in their times of need.

Most of us say we love our parents, and most of us really do. All we need to remind ourselves of that sacred emotion is to think back on the myriad good memories stored deep in our minds. Or to think about those silly occasions when we did truly dumb things and our parents got us through them with a good laugh and some good advice. Or to think about how we all laughed and hugged and celebrated special events and achievements. And the moments when we were afraid and they gave us comfort and confidence. And to remember how they worried about us and gave us advice we often ignored, and how they stood by us through our personal trials and tribulations as we crossed the invisible boundary between youth and adulthood.

Parenting Your Parents is about you. About what you will want and need to think through as you embark on a tumultuous journey of caring about and for your aging parents. Or about what you need to consider right now, because you haven't planned or prepared for the onslaught of challenges that surely will bear down on you with an intensity and weight you simply won't have anticipated.

Parenting Your Parents looks at what people just like you are facing and examines how everyone is coping. And it's rich with the thoughts, ideas, and advice of one of Canada's pre-eminent geriatric health care professionals, who provides counsel and support every year to hundreds of elderly people in need of expert insight.

Parenting Your Parents is also a book about hope. It demonstrates that you're not alone — that hundreds of thousands of us face similar challenges every day, everywhere. We're all in this together, only we tend not to think of it that way. Most of us think that what we're facing is a singular, personal journey into the unknown. But the reality is that we all share a common responsibility of providing our parents with the love, care, support, affection, and attention that they need and that we can deliver if we set our minds to it and plan now.

This is a book of hope because it shares stories of others who are dealing with the same kinds of problems you are facing, or will face; because we help you plan for what you will have to consider and do at some point in time; and because it encourages you to think about the future and how to deal with it, rather than simply wait to be blindsided by the course of events.

Finally, *Parenting Your Parents* is a practical book that provides you with an extensive listing of organizations across the country that offer the kind of support and services you may need for your parents — or for yourself.

But it is not a book with all the answers. Seldom is anyone doing it all the "right" way. What we bring you in this book are first-hand experiences, learned lessons to share, and many observations about the trauma, turmoil, and challenges we're all facing or about to face.

As you read these words — at this very moment — a parent, somewhere, is in dire need of medical attention. And, somewhere, a parent is dying. And, somewhere else, a parent is about to fall and break a hip. And so it goes. So the story of our lives unfolds. None of us with parents is exempt from the process and consequences of the passage of time. It is time to repay the profound debts we owe our parents who so much wanted us to forge and find our own good life.

Two days ago, my mother leaned on a dining room chair; it toppled and she fell. She was in pain all that night — especially her left arm — and the next morning the young woman who helps my parents took my mother to the emergency department of North York General Hospital. The X-ray showed a broken left wrist. Today, my mother is in bed with a cast to her elbow. She's being a real sport about it, but clearly she's in great discomfort and some pain. And she's confused by this new and unwanted experience. She doesn't yet know how to manage it. And she's looking for a lot of comforting support.

This morning I charged through the client work I had to do and then went to see her. She'd had a very bad night. So had my father. They both looked haggard. After all, my father, who has never fallen through all these years, had slipped in his bedroom just three weeks ago and fractured his left arm. He was in a cast from shoulder to fingers for ten long, dreary days. His cast came off only five days before my mother's fall. They'd just begun to return to their routines, and now they are faced with her being in a cast for an estimated five weeks.

So I went to visit and help. I first helped my mother get out of bed, and it pained me to watch how uncertain she was when she finally stood and took a few tentative, wobbly steps. Determined, she walked the length of the hallway to the dining room, and then she wanted to get back into bed. We got all that done while my father finished dressing, and by that time he wanted to sit down for a short rest. And while he was calling me with questions about this and that, my mother was talking to me about her condition. But since both are now hard of hearing, they were competing for my attention without either knowing it. After dashing back and forth to listen — and respond — to both of them, I got them as settled and comfortable as possible.

Then I went grocery shopping for them. I looked for and selected things they really like, and especially those that are easily prepared. Knowing that my mother wouldn't be able to do much in the way of cooking or serving meals, I decided to make sure they were stocked with things I knew my father liked a lot and could easily prepare, and things I knew my mother liked to munch on. After showing my father what I had bought and storing everything where it belonged, I told my mother about my purchases so she'd know, and then I helped her up again and got her to sit at the kitchen table for a meal their helper was preparing.

Then I left for the day. This evening I called to see how they were doing. My mother said they were tired, but stable. Tomorrow, I will go to see them and help as best I can for a while. But now I will work on client projects in order to catch up and stay on top of what I need to do for our business. It's close to midnight. But I'm juggling. Balancing my work world responsibilities with what I feel are my responsibilities to my parents.

My partner in life and work, Gail, understands and is hugely support-ive. But it's evident that if we didn't have our own business, caring for my parents would be immensely difficult, if not impossible. As it is, we aren't as productive in our business as we could be, because for the past few months I've been spending about fifteen to twenty hours a week helping my parents. Gail's sensitivity stems from losing her mother to an obscure disease at an early age — in her mid-sixties — more than a decade ago, and from losing her father to cancer four years ago. Those painful events are still vivid in our minds and hearts, but even more so in hers.

Having our own business gives me the freedom and room to help my parents in a way that wouldn't be possible if I had a traditional corporate job. In fact, I remember seeing a news story that said research has shown that many people are losing opportunities for career advancement because they're passing on training and being overlooked for promo-tions since they need time off for parent care. That reminds me how long it took to get enlightened child care policies in the workplace, and it makes me wonder how long it will be before organizations become respectful and sensitive to the reality of the other end of life's spectrum and allow room in the working day for eldercare.

Meanwhile, Gail and I are living in a perpetual state of anticipation, concern, and, frankly, fear. Fear of the inevitable. Fear that we didn't do something we should have done. Concern that my parents have all they need to be comfortable. And the sad anticipation that at some point, some day, one of them will die, and we will need the strength and ability to help the surviving one, and ourselves, to face the future.

The lesson to be learned? There's nothing pretty about any of this. It's the drama of life and death. It's why we're here on the good planet Earth as human beings with emotions and values and passion.

It starts with the aging of our parents. It progresses through various stages of their needs and the need for our support. It creates demands for which, for the most part, we're unprepared. Every step of the way, we come to realize how fragile we are and how frightening this journey really is.

And on this journey, nothing is clear or certain. Nothing is a given. There are no definite timelines or rules. Only, perhaps, that as the aging children of aging parents, we have a very difficult and critical and loving role to play. It's all about obligations and expectations — those of our parents and of ourselves.

It's all about finding coping mechanisms that allow us to do the best we can, to make our parents' lives as comfortable and meaningful as possible, while still managing to have a life of our own.

It's all about learning how to help, but also about the limits of help without feeling guilt.

It's all about compassion and caring, and finding a way and means, while not losing ourselves in the process, to support those very parents who for so long did so much for us, and who now need us to do so much for them.

And that's precisely what we explore in this book. We give you a roadmap to build your confidence — to show you that you're far from being alone on what you may have thought was a lonely passage into the realm of caring for and helping your parents through their time of need.

Bart Mindszenthy

THE ROCKY ROAD OF RESPONSIBILITY

K elly, a friend of many years, leans across the pub table with a beer in hand and says, "All our lives, we have this relationship with our parents where we expect them to be there, and we just don't talk about what would happen if things really change, if they're not there in the same way, and what we need to do, and how we plan for that." I ponder Kelly's thought. He's right. We all face the same dilemma.

We talk some more about parents. How they're so much a part of our lives. How we both know them, and don't know them. How we're both close, but not. How we think we'll be able to manage the process of supporting them, but when push comes to shove, there are so many unknowns along the course of life that we often don't know what to do or the best way to do it.

We're not talking about parents dying. We're talking about parents at the end game of their lives, when their mental and physical capabilities are in rapid and steady decline. When, seemingly from one day to the next, we — the children of our parents — find that we're cast into the uncharted and unwelcome role of caregivers to our parents.

A few beers later, Kelly and I agree that our world is different. The old world was one where families were generally closer where the care of elderly fathers and mothers was easier just two generations ago because usually the woman didn't work outside the home and was a mainstay in helping aging parents while juggling responsibilities with children. But, for better or for worse, that's not today's world. Women take a much more active part in the world of work outside the home, even while continuing to carry much of the responsibility of home-making and child rearing. And, often, they are the primary if not exclusive caregivers to their parents and sometimes even their in-laws. However, more and more, sons and sons-in-law are taking on these roles as well, and the world of work and new family structures are undergoing many confusing, contemporary changes.

We also talk about how aging parents have demands that are difficult to meet. As they age, our parents seem to simultaneously push and pull: push us away with outlandish views, and pull us closer with their needs and increasingly frequent voyages into their precious memories of the past in which we play a dominant role. For, as they age, our parents seem to find comfort in the distant past and like to recall the many good and funny and emotional experiences we shared those many years ago.

As Kelly and I ponder these thoughts, I can't help but think about what hundreds of friends and acquaintances have told me over the past months since Michael and I started working on this book. All of them, when learning that we were working on a book called *Parenting Your Parents*, have been amazingly open in wanting to share their own experiences, worries, challenges, and trepidation. Frankly, I'm astounded by the candour of people who seem keen to talk about how they're trying to help their parents while managing their own day-to-day lives.

People's stories range from the sad to the humorous, and include weird and wonderful anecdotes about the real-life situations they're all facing. What they all have in common is the commitment to support their parents in any way they can, and the fact that doing so isn't easy or comfortable.

The very next day after my evening out with Kelly, I get a call from Brian, a friend in Vancouver. During the course of our conversation, Brian talks about the difficulty of dealing with his parents as they age.

Both are eighty-six years old, Brian reports, and it's so very difficult to listen to them and to help them. His father, who is blind, is very demanding. He wants meals at a certain time; he wants attention and help in a certain way. He wants many things, and expects to get them when he thinks it's best for him. Brian's mother has been coping as best she can, but not long ago she simply collapsed from exhaustion. Brian had her admitted to a hospital and then made sure she stayed there for a week just to get a rest and a break from being the principal caregiver to her husband, while no one was principal caregiver to her. The week helped, but Brian is worried that his mother may collapse again given the strain of supporting her husband with no relief in sight.

Then I talk to good friend and business associate Judith in Toronto. Her father died two years ago, and last year, after a lot of researching, she located a good seniors' home for her mother. Now her mother is happy with her setting. Judith visits regularly, helps her mother with her financial matters, and shares a special time once a week over a late afternoon cocktail and dinner. This is a time they both relish, savour, and look forward to, and a time when Judith can carefully observe her mother to catch any changes that need to be considered.

Judith and her mother are fortunate because they can lead relatively normal lives and share the best with each other. Yet Judith is cautious and careful, making certain that her mother is both comfortable and secure on all counts, while fully cognizant that down the line her mother's condition will deteriorate. What Judith seems to be doing right is planning ahead and staying in close touch with her mother and the caregivers at the retirement home where her mother lives.

Shortly afterwards, my long-time friend Françoise, now living in the Eastern Townships southeast of Montreal, calls to check in. During our conversation, she tells me that her aging father is still as unpredictable as ever, and relates how frustrating it is to visit him on days when he either can't or elects not to remember what's happening or why. Her father has been drinking more than he should for some time now, and no matter how hard Françoise and her sister try, they can't get him away from the habit, which sometimes causes embarrassing and difficult family get-togethers.

This conversation makes me think of my partner's father, who was highly unpredictable and loved his independence until his bout with cancer. I remember how Gail's family dealt with his death. How for many months we watched him slide ever lower, all the way fighting the concept of death, using every ounce of his energy to stay lucid and alive. All this, while Gail and her brother arranged for every needed in-home service available to make their father as comfortable as possible while his pain grew day by day.

And there are so many others, all with a common concern, fear, confusion, and anxiety: how to support, help, and deal with aging parents. How to do what's right, while balancing a demanding life with their own families in a world that's moving too fast, and where the rules are changing all the time.

Many of us feel enormous love and gratitude for what our parents have given to us and for the many sacrifices they made throughout their lives for us. Some immigrated so that their children could live better lives. Some worked at more than one job to secure their children a more comfortable life. Others took risks at work in order to improve their standard of living so that their children could study and find good jobs. Now it's our turn to care for them as they have cared for us: with love and devotion, even when the struggles and the challenges are sometimes overwhelming as we try to live our lives while we help our parents live their own lives to the fullest.

All the people I have talked to have poignant, intimate, emotional stories that are embedded in a not-too-distant past that is still vivid in their mind's eye. All of them wonder what they might have done differently to make the outcome better, more fulfilling, and less painful. And all of them regret that somehow, in some way, they couldn't have made it easier on everyone.

Listening hard, I realize that a consistent set of observations and frustrations emerges:

- Parents have high expectations of receiving attention and all the things they think they want, and low tolerance for those events and things they want to ignore or avoid.
- Parents usually choose to remember being right and doing the right thing.
- Parents think we, their children, stay children, no matter what our age.
- Parents will try to protect us even while expecting us to help when necessary.
- Parents don't want to lose their influence over us.
- Parents don't want to lose their sense of independence or dignity.
- Parents who are still together will defend each other with passion, even if they know that one of them has erred.
- Parents who have problems in their relationship with each other continue to have those problems even as they age; sometimes the issues become caricatures of those they experienced in their younger years.
- Parents, as they age and become more fragile, will rationalize their thinking and actions for fear of losing personal and family control.
- Parents see the world as they want, and there's nothing we can do to change that.
- Parents usually don't want to admit until it's too late that they need to rely on us, at which point we're usually frustrated and unsure of how we can deliver the support they need.

So it's not an easy challenge that we, the children of our parents, face when we become by default their caregivers. Their wants and needs are demanding, and our ability to deliver is usually limited by time, resources, and priorities. Even when we want to give more, we are often in a conflict with the other demands on our lives — from our spouses, our children, and our work. There is an ongoing battle within us between meeting the demands of our daily lives and meeting our parents' needs.

But, as Michael cautions throughout this book, this continuing internal battle can lead to problems if we don't measure carefully what we are realistically able to do, even when taking all the necessary steps to succeed. If we are not careful in how we pace and control what we are able to do, we can set ourselves up for terrible failure and risk undermining our own well-being and ability to care successfully for our parents. If we don't balance all the demands of our lives, we'll likely short-circuit ourselves along the way. We'll suffer mentally, and maybe even physically.

And if that happens, we won't be much good to anyone — our spouse, our children, our parents, our employers, or ourselves. That's why we need to step back, assess, and take inventory of what we need to do to plan for and implement a sound, firm, logical strategy for helping our parents effectively and lovingly.

What we're into, in fact, is a delicate, difficult phase of our lives. There are no easy answers or magical solutions. The reality is that we'll all suffer, but at times we will also grow as we find new strength in our accomplishments. We need to try to maximize the small satisfactions and minimize the anguish and pain that often occur as part of the aging process of our parents. At the end of the day, we should be able to say that we did what we could and were fortunate enough to have had the opportunity to care for our aging parents, through all the challenges and difficulties, and be better children and adults from the experience.

Another reality is that, despite the challenges, we're expressing love and affection for our parents. We're showing them the respect and support they need and have every right to expect. We're simply balancing the scorecard of life. Because when we sit back dispassionately and take a lifelong inventory, chances are we'll find that in all the years since we were born, our parents did an awful lot for us. No doubt, we can all remember bad experiences. But the good experiences, and the good intent, almost always far outweigh the bad.

Caring for our parents can be tough and trying, yet if we really do love them for who they are and what they've tried to do for us, then it's a natural, healthy, and important commitment to make and take seriously.

And no matter how hard things get — how trying — what must drive us is the wish and will to give our parents the comfort and dignity they deserve. So while our heads may stay pragmatic, our hearts will drive us to help them through the most difficult, demanding times. Because, bluntly put, that's the way life works. And that's what each one of us with children hope will be the case when we're in need — even if we don't admit it.

CONTROL:

Laying on the Guilt Trip

For whatever reason, some parents find it necessary to induce a sense of guilt in their children, and sometimes even their grandchildren, making relations difficult and sometimes strained. Careful planning is necessary to defuse this very delicate situation.

THE CHALLENGE

Beth and Lloyd Thurmont are eighty-three and eighty-six years old, respectively. They have three children — Darrin, who is fifty-eight; Donna, fifty-six; and Cameron, fifty-four. Beth and Lloyd live in a retirement home on the outskirts of Orangeville, Ontario.

Darrin, a chartered accountant, lives with his family in Brampton (a forty-five-minute drive away). He and his wife, Betty, have four children: thirty-year-old twin sisters Tracy and Tammy; Tom, who is twenty-eight and lives in London, Ontario, with his wife, Angela, and their four children; and twenty-six-year-old Terry, who lives in Toronto with her lesbian partner.

Donna's marriage fell apart two years ago when her husband announced he was leaving for another job in Vancouver and wanted to start life over again. They have one child, Arthur, who at thirty-eight goes from job to job and city to city, still looking for a career path that suits him. Donna lives in a downtown Toronto bachelor apartment and works as a paralegal at a large law firm.

Cameron lives in Berlin, Germany, where he's been working as a freelance artist for the past five years. He enjoys his work and where he lives immensely. Single and unattached, Cameron loves roaming around Europe and has been back to Canada only twice to visit family and friends. He does call his parents about twice a month, and he sends them email messages through his brother, Darrin.

Lloyd has been in ailing health for some years and is visited regularly by a nurse arranged through Ontario's Community Care Access Centre services, as well as by a physiotherapist who helps him exercise his severely arthritic legs and arms. Beth is in relatively good health, except for Type 2 diabetes, controlled by medication, and a weight problem she's had for decades.

Beth longs to have her children pay more attention to her and Lloyd and to see more of her grandchildren. No matter how much attention her family pays to her and Lloyd, for Beth it's not enough. She believes that in their old age she and her husband are entitled to as much of their children's and grandchildren's time as they want and need.

In fact, in the past few years Beth has been exerting a steadily increasing level of control over her family by playing on their fears and instilling feelings of guilt. This has led to instances of both capitulation and confrontation among her children. Sometimes they've given in to the pressures placed on them, and sometimes they've had violent verbal battles. But most often, they've acquiesced in order to keep the peace and because their father always asks them to bear their mother's insecurities and to put up with her needs.

But now Beth's claims and attacks are more frequent and her needs more intense. She often calls with pleas for a quick appearance by one of her children because, she claims, Lloyd is desperate to see Darrin or Donna — usually a surprise to Lloyd, who is content to watch movies and read magazines most of the time. And every so often she attacks Donna for failing in her marriage and causing embarrassment and grief for the whole family. Meanwhile, she alleges that Cameron rarely visits because he is selfish and has elected to escape his family responsibilities and that he lives a decadent life far away while everyone else is close to home and willing to help. And Darrin, she says, is guilty of putting his family before his parents because he visits only for an hour or so once or twice a week.

Beth is scathing in her views of her grandchildren, who, she alleges, are only waiting to inherit the small fortune she and Lloyd have managed to save through years of back-breaking work. (The truth is that Beth and Lloyd are not very well off, and their three children actually contribute to offset the cost of their living in the retirement home.) She often tells her children that they, like her grandchildren, would be smart to be nicer to her and Lloyd or they may lose their inheritance in favour of some worthy cause. And ever since Beth discovered that Terry is a lesbian, she regularly harasses Darrin and Betty about it, telling them that if she were Terry's mother, this would never have happened. Terry, not surprisingly, has refused to see her grandmother for several years. Beth's other grandchildren tend to avoid any interaction with her, although they do confess to their parents that they would like to visit Lloyd alone, if that were possible.

No matter what responses her children give, Beth counters all of them with emotional outpourings and claims of feeling unwell or rejected. She works very hard at making all her children feel guilty in different ways.

For Beth's birthday in January, Darrin came to collect her and Lloyd and took them to his Brampton home, where Betty had prepared a lavish dinner. All four of Darrin and Betty's children attended, as did Donna. But by midway through dinner everyone was miserable, as Beth spent considerable time telling stories about how during the past year she and Lloyd had been disappointed and hurt by their children's insensitivity and their grandchildren's poor behaviour. The event turned into a painful experience for all of them, and at one point Donna got into a bitter exchange with her mother that left all of them hurt and embarrassed.

When she hasn't slept well for a couple of nights, or when she's feeling especially lonely and depressed, Beth calls her children and becomes agitated and confrontational, and the content of her message is almost always the same: "What are you doing for me today?" Now, it's reaching the point where her children want to rebel and find ways to contain her outrageous claims, accusations, and anger.

Meanwhile, Lloyd continues to distance himself from the tension the family is feeling. For whatever reason, when he does talk to his children, it's always in a remote way that seems to imply his lack of interest in his wife's needs and intensity. Lloyd, when he does see one of his children or talk to one of his grandchildren, usually discusses some movie or television special he's seen or an article he's read in *Reader's Digest*. And when he talks about Beth and her behaviour, it's usually in a very passive way, simply asking the family to be understanding and to ignore her accusations.

But the reality is that Darrin and Donna are having an increasingly difficult time coping with their mother's attitude and outbursts. And since they can't detect any certain signs of mental illness or any other problem, they are confused and frustrated. They relay their impressions to Cameron, who says he just isn't close enough to be able to pass judgment.

Darrin recently spoke to his parents' family physician, who said that there doesn't seem to be anything wrong with Beth. In fact, she seems relatively well, generally upbeat, and positive about her life, but she has expressed concerns that her children and grandchildren are ignoring Lloyd, and this she finds hurtful and wrong. She told the doctor that Lloyd suffers as a result and that, in turn, she's stressed. The doctor told Darrin that Beth did volunteer that she misses more interaction with her children and grandchildren, and that she believes all of them would just as soon see her and Lloyd dead and gone so they wouldn't have to care about them.

Darrin, in sharing this information with Donna and Cameron, also tells them that he feels their parents' doctor sympathizes with their mother's sense of being wronged. He tells them he's concerned that the doctor is, for whatever reason, biased in her favour, and that as a result he's not being as helpful as he should be in assessing her and possibly prescribing some kind of medication to manage her moods.

THE HEALTH CARE PROFESSIONAL'S POINT OF VIEW

This is the kind of difficult family dynamic that can either lead to further family disruption, with a permanent legacy of hurt and guilt, or bring a family together and demonstrate how robust they are in dealing with difficult situations. Most families at times have to face trying situations that may test the very fabric of family ties. Whether the issue involves illness, death, terrible financial situations, or complex family dynamics, there are ways of reaching resolutions so that irremediable damage does not occur.

We will work on the assumption that there is nothing wrong with Beth medically that can account for her increasing need for family attention and that, therefore, her behaviour is merely a manifestation of her underlying personality. Even though the family physician may not believe there is anything wrong with her, it may be worthwhile for a family spokesperson to speak to the doctor and question whether, indeed, something underlying might be going on. Sometimes conditions such as depression or early dementia result in peculiar exaggerations of personality. The family physician can address this possibility by probing for symptoms and conducting mental-status tests. If the physician is sure that what is going on is not related to an underlying clinical condition, then Beth has to be dealt with as a full participant in whatever process might be developed to help resolve this increasingly tense and potentially destructive situation.

To assist the family and Beth and Lloyd, a two-part process can be implemented. First, the children, especially the two in Ontario, need to get some help in sorting through this very challenging situation. If this is not done in some cohesive fashion, the result could be terrible alienation of the various members of the family that is likely to have long-lasting effects on the family structure. It is important that the grandchildren who live in the vicinity also take part in the process, as the patterns of family interaction, the value put on relationships, and the ability to deal with difficulty are often measures of a family's strength for the present and the future.

One approach is to find a social worker (or some other family counsellor) who is experienced in dealing with issues of family dynamics. It is important to define who the key players will be in any family meetings that take place initially to try to provide a framework for the issues, problems, and options. But, even for those who do not actually attend family sessions, there must be consistent communication so that everyone is on board with the approach. This is an opportunity for all the children to address the issues and, if at all possible, to be consistent with the approach to their parents (and grandparents).

Assuming that such family counselling takes place, the second part of the process is to have a clear discussion with Beth and Lloyd about what is going on. There may be a number of ways of doing this, including having the key members of the family meet with Beth and Lloyd alone (not too many in the first meeting, but clearly representing the consensus of the family) to explain the enormous difficulties that everyone is facing.

It makes sense to begin a meeting of this sort with a clear statement of the love, devotion, and commitment the family has for their parents, and to explain that it might not be possible to carry out their own complex lives and at the same time respond to Beth's every whim and need.

Of course at this point, it is possible that Beth may become very upset or angry at being "ganged up on," and she may not want any further part of the discussions. If this happens, it would be time for one person, perhaps Darrin, to speak to his mother again and continue with the same message: "We love you and Dad, and we want only the best for you, but…," laying out the difficulties that everyone is facing. It must be made clear to Beth that insulting her children and grand-children has the opposite effect to the one she hopes to achieve.

It might be suggested to Beth and Lloyd (or to Beth alone if that seems preferable) that she join a few of the family members to meet with the counsellor. If she agrees, that is a major step forward. If she rejects that offer, it may still be possible to work with her and Lloyd to find an acceptable and agreeable common ground.

Arrangements that sometimes work in such situations include developing a rotation system of who will visit or communicate with whom on a regular basis. There may be some need to increase the interaction of the family with Lloyd and Beth, but rather than that interaction being on an on-call basis, the family could put together an outline of what can and cannot be done reasonably within clearly defined limits.

Someone should make it clear that there are no financial expectations from Beth and Lloyd, and if, indeed, the children are paying for some of the expenses, this can be pointed out. Most important, it must be related to Beth, either by a family member (or two) or by a counsellor, that her recriminations and accusations are disruptive and may ultimately cause the family network and ties to unravel. That would be the worst outcome possible, because eventually Beth and Lloyd may have needs that will require a great deal of devotion and time, and an enormous sense of guilt may follow the family members for years to come.

Family dynamics is among the most difficult issues to challenge. But the children and grandchildren have to come to terms with the long-haul implications of the decisions they make. Families are not replaced by other entities, and it is worth the investment to try to salvage whatever relationships exist for the immediate situation and for the future. There are ways of learning how not to react to hurtful words when it is clear that the result will be counterproductive. There are ways for Beth's family to remind her consistently that her family loves her but that she must find better ways to help them carry out their love than trying to bully them into it.

SURGERY:

Weighing the Odds

Surgery at any age can be traumatic, but for the elderly there are special issues and considerations. Weighing priorities and planning recovery is a complex and demanding process that requires careful consideration.

THE CHALLENGE

Lee Ann Bowater is seventy-six and a widow. Her husband, Martin, died four years ago after suffering several heart attacks. She lives alone in a one-bedroom apartment in Halifax, and while she still mourns Martin's death, she has moved on with her life. Lee Ann has several friends, and they try to get together at least once a week for tea and talk.

Lee Ann's daughter, Sylvia, is an elementary school teacher. She's fifty-two years old and lives in Dartmouth with her husband, Gerry, who works long hours managing a car rental outlet in downtown Halifax. Sylvia and Gerry have two children: Jay, age twenty-eight, and Linda, age nineteen. Jay moved to Moncton three years ago to work in a call centre, and Linda lives at home as she continues her education at a local college.

Lee Ann's son, David, is forty-seven years old and lives in Calgary, where he works as an analyst for an oil company. He divorced two years ago and lives in an apartment with his common-law partner, Mary, whom Lee Ann has never met.

Both children are in close contact with Lee Ann, especially Sylvia, who lives only twelve kilometres away and visits her mother every other day. As well, once every two weeks Gerry picks up Lee Ann to take her to their home for dinner. David calls from Calgary at least once a week to talk to his mother for a few minutes, and he tries to visit at least once a year.

Lee Ann relishes visits from her daughter, and she tries hard to be a loving, non-intrusive grandmother to Jay and Linda, although she considers both to be somewhat spoiled. However, she works very hard at keeping those feelings to herself, and she spends most of the time during Sylvia's visits asking about her teaching and Gerry's work.

Lee Ann is relatively sound in body and mind. She is short and a bit overweight, but not so much that it's a problem. In fact, since Martin's death, she has shown a surprisingly strong sense of independence and has learned to manage her finances so that Gerry needs to spend only an hour a month reviewing her bank statements.

Five years ago Lee Ann had surgery for cataracts in both eyes. This was a low-risk, high-benefit proposition that allowed her to see well again and resume a relatively normal lifestyle. In fact, she found she could once again play canasta with her friends.

Now, however, Lee Ann has developed a malignant tumour in her colon that is still relatively small but has the potential to grow and spread. Her doctor believes surgery will be required at some point. As well, she is in constant pain because of severe osteoarthritis in her left hip, and a hip replacement operation is the only certain way to help her with that condition.

Lee Ann's doctor is cautious about the prognosis, noting that while the operations are fairly routine, Lee Ann will need substantial support for a prolonged period of time afterward. The hip operation is not critical, but it would allow Lee Ann to walk and function more easily and would probably eliminate the pain with which she's living. The colon surgery, on the other hand, is more urgent because of the risk of the tumour spreading.

Lee Ann understands that she needs the colon surgery, and she also wants the hip replacement, but she is fearful of the two operations and the period of convalescence that would follow. It's clear that if either operation is to proceed, Lee Ann will require close, ongoing help and support during her recovery.

Sylvia knows that her mother would like to live with her and Gerry during her recovery. Gerry is against this idea because they live in a small house with two bedrooms, and they both work full-time. While he hasn't said no to the prospect of Lee Ann living with them, it is not an option he would happily embrace.

David has said that he wants to be supportive but that distance prevents him from doing much in terms of hands-on help.

Given Lee Ann's limited income, as well as the limited incomes of both Sylvia and David, there is no clear resolution to the question of how the family will support her.

The challenge for the family is how to help Lee Ann face two surgical procedures, both of which are necessary to give her a chance of survival and an improved quality of life. How can they help without disrupting their own equilibrium in an unacceptable way? The family faces several important issues. Should the colon surgery be performed first? If so, Lee Ann would require at least two or three weeks of in-home care. But where should she stay for that period of time? If she were to remain in her apartment, she would require professional home care services, as well as someone to live with her during her convalescence. Or, could Lee Ann stay with Sylvia and her family, or with David and his partner? Could David take a few weeks off and stay with his mother?

If the colon surgery is performed first and Lee Ann has a good recovery, then should the orthopedic surgery be undertaken to replace her left hip? And if so, when? Rehabilitation work would be necessary after the hip surgery, and that would mean Lee Ann would have to be taken for rehab sessions at least twice a week for several weeks.

Sylvia and Gerry have talked about what they could and should do. Their daughter, Linda, has made it clear that she won't have time to help because of her school and social commitments. Their son, Jay, is relatively independent but works long hours. Sylvia is concerned about any surgery taking place during the school year because she won't be able to take the kind of time off that would probably be required. And Gerry, given the nature of his job, can't be counted on for any extended level of support.

Sylvia has discussed the situation with her brother during the course of several telephone conversations. She's even suggested that David take his holidays and spend two weeks with their mother after the colon operation to help her. David listened to the case Sylvia presented but responded by saying that Mary was really counting on having their holidays together for a long-planned drive to tour the Grand Canyon and to spend time in Las Vegas. This has irritated Sylvia, but the siblings have stayed very polite with each other.

Lee Ann's doctor, in a recent telephone call with Sylvia, advised that while he wants to do some further tests, he believes the colon surgery will be imperative based on the steady growth of the tumour. He tells Sylvia that "sooner than later" is the way they should think about it.

THE HEALTH CARE PROFESSIONAL'S POINT OF VIEW

Lee Ann and her family have a few things to figure out, and a real examination of relationships and priorities is necessary in order for this situation to work well. It is worth dividing the issues into those that are mainly clinical and those that are related to the way the family feels they should and can support Lee Ann, who wants to remain independent, but who is facing some difficult challenges in the next little while.

When considering the clinical issues, the priority is likely going to be the removal of the colon tumour. Based on the information pro-vided, it appears that the tumour is still at a stage where if it is removed surgically, a good outcome is likely and Lee Ann should be able to function independently.

It is worth asking the surgeon if the surgery can be done in such a way that bowel function will be maintained and a colostomy (exit of bowel through the skin) will not be required. The answer will have a big impact on the type of care required immediately after the surgery and for the longer term following.

Also, the assumption is that the tumour will be contained and will not spread (metastasize) to other organs, so that the outlook over a longer period of time would be good. However, until the surgery is done it is hard to know whether further treatments such as radiation therapy might be required.

The family must understand that there is some urgency to the decision about the colon surgery and that they must find ways to support their mother through this emotionally and physically trying situation. Although Lee Ann may be holding herself together in face of what is probably a very frightening prospect, it appears that she does not want to be a burden on her family. This is the time for her children to find the means to rally around and support their mother, one way or another, within the resources, human and otherwise, that they have available.

They can look at the challenges in a few stages. The first is the immediate preparation for surgery, with its emotional and physical impacts. This is the time for everyone to find time and, in a co-operative fashion, to be there to bolster their mother (and grandmother).

Assuming that all goes well, the stages following surgery will be divided into the immediate post-operative phase and then a period of Lee Ann's reactivation and return to a normal functioning lifestyle. It is important for the family to explore what assistance is available for their mother's post-surgical care to help all of them cope in terms of time limitations. Although such assistance often does not completely replace the need for family, it can provide proper care for the patient while families carry on with their other responsibilities. Reactivation programs in long-term care facilities may be available in some jurisdictions, and home care options, providing nursing care and some homemaking, may be available as part of the health care program. These services may have to be supplemented through paid help in addition to whatever the family can weave together to support their mother in getting over the immediate post-operative and return-to-home period.

It would be worth exploring whether there are friends and neighbours available to give a little help. In fact, such help may very well be readily forthcoming and may pleasantly surprise the family and Lee Ann. Although the family may not want to impose on others, often neighbours and friends feel that helping out is one of the ways to demonstrate affection and caring, so the idea of asking for help should not be dismissed out of hand.

It's a real challenge to families when they have to interrupt their busy lives to deal with a family crisis. But everyone in the family has to step back and ask, "Do I want my mother [grandmother, mother-in-law, etc.] to survive this ordeal?" After all, family should take priority in times of difficulty, and major cancer surgery is just that kind of challenge.

Lee Ann's moving into Sylvia's home is probably not ideal given the cramped space, but if another arrangement cannot be made for the immediate period after surgery this option should be reconsidered. Families can usually find ways to come together during times of crisis, and Lee Ann's surgery should be considered to be precisely that: a crisis in the making. Most employers are understanding when there is a family illness, and it may be necessary for family members to get some extra time off to help look after Lee Ann at Sylvia and Gerry's home until she feels secure enough to return to her own home with some home care in addition to what her family can provide.

As for David, this is a time to test his relationships. It would seem reasonable to expect one's significant other to compromise on vacation plans if a family member's health is at stake. David's moving in with his mother for a week might make all the difference, with a little supplement from home care professionals and homemakers and input from other family members, including the grandchildren, in helping Lee Ann get over this difficult time. The way everyone comes together in this time of need will be a reflection of the fabric of this family. Anyone can be constructive and positive when there are no demands. It is during difficult times that a family's true strength is tested, and for Lee Ann's family, this is such a time.

If Lee Ann gets through the colon surgery without much difficulty, the issue of her hip should be a lesser challenge. First, if the colon surgery goes well, that experience should help Lee Ann and her family understand the steps necessary to negotiate the health care and home care systems. Second, there are often programs in place to assist in the rehabilitation process following major orthopaedic surgery.

It would be wise for Lee Ann to wait at least three months after the colon surgery to have the hip operation. This should give her ample time to regain her emotional and physical strength and her independence. If more time for recovery is required, then the hip surgery should be done later, as the urgency for it is not great.

Lee Ann's family should inquire whether or not in-patient rehabilitation exists. If it does, arrangements should be made after discussions with the orthopaedic surgeon and, if appropriate, the social service department of the hospital to make certain that the post-operative plan includes admission at an in-patient rehabilitation unit. If such an arrangement is possible (and it usually is), then Lee Ann's concerns about being a burden to her family and disrupting their lives change considerably. Following anywhere from four to six weeks on a rehabilitation unit, Lee Ann will in all likelihood be able to return home with minimal assistance.

Most rehabilitation programs provide some evaluation of the home setting and recommend or arrange for modifications to accommodate the patient's ability to function. If the hip replacement will make Lee Ann more independent than she was prior to surgery, it is likely that little, if anything, will have to be done to the home to meet her needs. However, some safety measures might be recommended, especially in the bathroom to make sure she can bathe safely with minimal risk of falling.

If Lee Ann and her children are concerned about Lee Ann being alone in her home, they can look into an emergency response system, such as Lifeline (see the Resource Directory at the back of the book), which allows individuals to call for help should they fall or injure themselves, providing a sense of security to clients and their families.

Illness poses a great challenge both to those affected by the illness and to their families. This is a special time for families to enrich their relationships and to demonstrate what they are willing and able to do for their loved one. It has to be a co-operative affair so that there is no lingering resentment that can cause hard feelings later. What better way to demonstrate affection to a parent in special need, even the most independent parent, than to help as an act of love and devotion? That is what families are all about.

ELDERTRAVEL:

Balancing Risks and Benefits

> *Travelling distances can be difficult*
> *these days even for the middle-aged,*
> *and all the more so for the elderly.*
> *Good intentions aside, any significant*
> *travel plans for the elderly must be*
> *carefully considered and, if they're to*
> *proceed, thoughtfully planned.*

THE CHALLENGE

Raul Rodregez is eighty years old. Born in Costa Rica, he moved to Canada in the early 1960s and two years later married Kate, a Canadian woman he had met a year earlier. They lived for some twenty years in Dartmouth, Nova Scotia, where Raul worked in the shipyards until he retired in 1984.

Kate gave birth to a daughter, Mandy, in 1966. They always were a close-knit family, and Kate's sudden death in an automobile accident some ten years ago devastated both Raul and Mandy.

Raul has a son, Ramon, from a previous marriage, who remained in Costa Rica and over the years built a successful restaurant business. They have always stayed in close touch; Raul would visit his homeland and son every two to three years, and Ramon has been coming to Canada three or four times a year to see his father since the mid-1990s, when Raul's health started to decline and after Kate had died. Ramon had never approved of his father's marriage to Kate, and although he'd met her only a few times, he'd always elected to dislike her, feeling strongly his father never should have remarried.

However, Ramon felt closer to Mandy. While he didn't consider Mandy a part of his true family, he did acknowledge that she worked hard and cared a great deal for his father. Yet whenever Ramon visited, he tended to dominate the relationships. Whether staying in his father's apartment or in a hotel during his visits, Ramon would make it clear that for the duration of his stay he would look after his father and that Mandy's presence wasn't necessary.

During the winter of 1999, Raul slipped and fell on an icy patch of sidewalk while walking to his nearby grocery store. He suffered what was diagnosed as a mild concussion, broke his right arm, and fractured his right pelvis. For weeks following his release from the hospital, Mandy spent several hours every day at his apartment caring for her father and spending time with him. She did all his shopping and prepared all his meals, while helping Raul adjust to using only his left arm and hand. Since Raul also was relatively immobile because of the fractured pelvis, Mandy helped him get out of bed in the morning and into bed at night until he was able to function again.

At her father's urging, she had called Ramon to report the incident and his condition. Ramon paid a hurried visit the following week and spent two days with his father. During the visit, he urged his father to return to Costa Rica. Ramon told Raul that his business was starting to prosper and that he would look after him much better than Mandy had been. He also reminded his father that in Costa Rica he could speak his native tongue, and assured him that he would find many new friends there. Raul appreciated his son's concerns and thoughts but told him that, for the time being, he felt he should stay in what had been his home city and homeland for some decades now.

Meanwhile, Mandy continued to look after her father. She arranged for special support services and physiotherapy sessions. She asked for and got a flex-hour work schedule from her employer, which made it easier for her to manage the added caregiving responsibilities she'd assumed.

For months following his fall, Raul seemed to be making real progress with his recovery. Then one morning, he lost his balance getting out his bathtub and fell. While he was diagnosed with nothing more severe than some bruises and a twisted ankle, somehow Raul seemed less able to recover. In fact, he required more attention and support.

Mandy arranged for in-home support and more physiotherapy sessions. But walking was now much more difficult for Raul, and he relied more and more on using a walker. Whenever Mandy took him outdoors, he was now in a wheelchair. His family physician ordered a battery of tests, and while the results were inconclusive, the doctor felt that Raul's initial fall could have caused more damage than originally suspected.

Over the following year, Raul became more and more reclusive and less and less certain of himself and his ability to walk.

During Ramon's last visit in January, he pressed his father to come to Costa Rica, at least a few weeks' visit. He predicted Raul would enjoy and benefit from the warm weather and change of scenery and that the visit would be good for his health. He insisted that any medical needs could be arranged easily and quickly.

Raul was more receptive this time. After a long winter, and feeling depressed about his condition, Raul told Mandy that perhaps a few weeks in his homeland would be good for him. Mandy couldn't disagree more. She challenged her father and Ramon, telling them that her father needed special care and that she had worked hard to arrange for him to get that care on a regular basis. She said that while the climate might be wonderful, there were just too many unknowns, and the possible risks outweighed the benefits.

While her father wavered and became indecisive, Ramon became all the more adamant. He argued passionately that his father had a right to go home and enjoy himself. He told Mandy that there was nothing she did that he couldn't do for his father, and that he was now financially well off and could arrange for anything that might be needed.

Mandy didn't know what to think or do. On the one hand, she loved her father and worried about his health and well-being. On the other hand, she started to wonder if she might be overreacting, and questioned herself about how much of her feelings were driven by Ramon's domineering behaviour. She was now confused and uncertain, but she felt a nagging concern about the dangers of such a major trip for her father at his age and in his condition.

THE HEALTH CARE PROFESSIONAL'S POINT OF VIEW

Travelling can present many problems and challenges for an older person — even when for a simple vacation. When the travel situation is more complex, as in this case, it is important to examine all the issues and implications of the travel itself, as well as the stay in the faraway place.

In this particular situation, the issues go way beyond the trip and revolve around the relationship between Ramon and Mandy and the way each sees the relationship to his/her father. The child who flies in periodically from a faraway place often has a very disruptive impact on the family that is struggling to keep things together, especially when a frail parent's immediate caregiver is struggling to find ways to meet his many medical and psychosocial needs. Whether from a true sense of devotion or from the need to be seen as being important and to be "doing something," these fly-in-and-fly-out children may cause havoc to arrangements carefully put together for the ailing and needy parent.

The first thing that has to happen before Raul goes on a trip to Costa Rica, for however long, is for Mandy and Ramon to find a way to agree on how Raul's long-term needs will be met by the two of them. Only then should the trip to Costa Rica be contemplated. It is also very unfair to try to direct the decision to Raul, who clearly is caught between his two children and would like to please both of them in addition to wanting to feel better. Mandy and Ramon have inadvertently put an unnecessary burden on their father and they should be taking steps to eradicate that uncomfortable experience. Their mutual priority should be the care and well-being of their father. They must put aside their own needs, even the ones couched as concern for their father. Ramon would like his father in Costa Rica for a number of reasons, but one might very well be so that he can demonstrate to his friends and family just how much he cares for his father, something he cannot do from afar.

Mandy may be acting in an overprotective manner, but much of that is probably based on suspicions of her half-brother's motivations and of his ability to take care of Raul should things not go smoothly. The real challenge for Mandy is to approach Ramon on general terms regarding their mutual care of their father. It probably would be worthwhile for Mandy to find a way to speak to Ramon openly and tell him that she is not necessarily opposed to Raul visiting Costa Rica for a short period, but that the trip must take place within a framework of a plan for the present and future of which they are both a part. The benefits would be that their father could finally feel comfortable knowing that the two of them have found a way to bridge their differences, which is something that a parent always wants. Ramon may not be aware of just how trying their lack of closeness has been for Raul, and anything that might make him feel better would be very important to him in these waning days of his life.

It might even be worthwhile to pursue whether Mandy could join her father on the trip to Costa Rica and be involved in his time there. That would probably be very meaningful for Raul and also possibly improve the relationship between Mandy and Ramon. It would then frame the trip differently — going from Ramon's arrangements for his father to his children's attempt to improve Raul's state of mind. Even if Mandy cannot stay for the whole trip, going on the flight and staying a few days to help get things settled would be beneficial if it could be arranged.

As for the trip itself, there are certain basic principles that should be kept in mind when frail seniors undertake longer trips, especially by air. Some of the factors that should be considered include the medical implications of travelling and being far away from the normal professional caregivers, the need for adequate insurance that can be counted on to cover unanticipated illness, the actual travel itself and its trials and tribulations, and the expected benefits of being in another place for a period of time.

The Medical Condition

One should not travel if a medical condition exists that requires frequent monitoring and has resulted in repeated, unexpected admissions to hospitals or emergency rooms. Most insurance companies will not cover individuals with such uncertain medical conditions. One guide insurance companies often use, sometimes erroneously, is whether changes to medications have occurred during a previously defined period (often ninety days). This guide sometimes does not make medical sense, as in the case of the discontinuation of a medication that is no longer necessary or a decrease in dosage because of better outcomes of an already established treatment. The reasons for any changes, especially positive ones, should be documented by the physician to make sure that, should something happen, there is a good sound explanation available that would not imply increased risk during the trip.

The risk of not being covered is potentially huge medical bills, especially, but not exclusively, from illness that occurs while outside the country. In Raul's case, considering his fragility and instability, it is very likely that adequate medical insurance to cover the trip will not be available. To travel without such insurance is financially very risky.

The Travel Itself

The trip itself might pose many problems and barriers, especially with the very long waits at airports due to heightened security. This might be a problem for frail, elderly individuals such as Raul. Problems with behaviour or potential agitation may also be reasons not to attempt to fly, as they are difficult to deal with on a plane and not fair to other passengers. For someone who has severe urinary urgency or incontinence, it's probably best not to fly at all; we all know how long the wait can be to use a washroom on an airplane. If there are problems in walking and falls might occur, it would be best to let the airline know beforehand so that arrangements can be made to provide shuttling from the check-in counter to the gate to avoid long walks. If Raul needs a wheelchair, for instance, that has to be arranged in advance with both airports. It is important to make sure that all necessary supplies, including medications, continence supplies, and, if there is a risk, a change of clothes, are easily accessible.

Benefits of Destination

The benefits of the trip should be weighed carefully. There are several important factors to consider: Will the trip be a vacation that will improve the person's sense of well-being? Can the trip be arranged so that it is safe? Will it relieve the person of having to face a bad winter? Will it reunite the person with a loved one? It is always necessary to make sure that there will be appropriate support and supervision to decrease potential danger. How necessary medical services will be provided and by whom, as well as who should be contacted in case of an emergency, must be determined before travel. In Raul's case, Ramon may be able to make many of these arrangements, because rather than the trip being a vacation in an unknown destination, it is in some ways a visit to a place of friends and family who should be able to provide the necessary supports once Raul arrives.

Travel is not as easy as it once was. With good planning many people can travel safely and enjoy the benefits of warmer climates, especially during our harsh Canadian winters. If the warmer climate is part of the rationale for this trip, then Ramon has to find a way to discuss openly with Mandy and if possible Raul all the implications of the trip. Maybe it can work, and indeed it might provide a lift to Raul's spirits and result in some improvement in the relationship between Mandy and Ramon. If there is such a chance, it might be worth the effort and potential risk. If not, and the trip might lead to further conflict and put Raul at unnecessary risk, perhaps it should be rejected as a viable option.

INDEPENDENCE:

Helping Parents Live Their Lives

Sometimes in their zeal to help and protect their parents, children add to their discomfort by making decisions that may be well intentioned but actually serve to disrupt tried and true lifestyles. The result is increased family tension and parental angst.

THE CHALLENGE

Ivan and Sophie Bogdonovich immigrated to Canada in 1948. Their eventual arrival here is a story in itself. During the depths of World War II, Ivan, who had been unwillingly conscripted into the Soviet army, was injured and judged unfit for further service. He was, however, assigned to work in a factory several hundred kilometres from his village. Two months before the end of the war, after nearly a year at the factory, he managed to escape, work his way back to his village, and reunite for one night with his family and wife.

Under the deep cover of the next night, he and his young wife, Sophie, left their native village in the Ukraine with only the clothes on their backs and a satchel full of food. They managed to reach the Austrian boarder just as the war ended, and they were two of the first few to be accepted into an Austrian refugee camp where they were interned for three years. They applied to both the United States and Canada for refugee status and were eventually linked through the Red Cross with a sponsor in Red Deer, Alberta. The sponsor was a distant relative who agreed to help them settle in Canada.

Ivan is now in his late seventies and Sophie is in her mid-seventies. (No one is certain of their ages, and no birth record has ever been found.) They're in fairly good health but starting to show signs of forgetfulness.

They have two sons: Boris, forty-nine, who was born in the Austrian refugee camp just months before the family came to Canada, and Bob, forty-one, who was born in Red Deer. Both brothers left home some twenty years ago and now live in Montreal. Because the brothers are close to each other and comfortable with their lives in Montreal, they decided that to best help their parents, they should move them to a retirement home close to them.

At the time of this decision, neither parent really wanted to leave Red Deer, where they had a number of friends and an active social life. They were well known in the community because, from the mid-1950s to just two years ago, they had operated a popular diner known for its spicy cabbage rolls, various potato soups, and other ethnic dishes. But Boris and Bob were persistent. During their annual visits and weekly telephone calls, the brothers made their case and finally convinced their parents that they should move to Montreal.

Nine months later, Ivan and Sophie sold their home, shipped their belongings ahead, and a week later took the train to Montreal. They had been to Montreal a handful of times during the past fifteen years to visit their sons, but they knew only a little about the city, which they considered to be somewhat intimidating in comparison to comfortably sized Red Deer. But as they got older, they also longed to be closer to their sons, and they knew of no other way than moving to make that possible.

Boris and Bob, who really are close to each other and very fond of their parents and proud of what they have done with their lives, were determined to make the move a good one. After considerable searching, they found a small but attractive one-bedroom apartment for their parents, which they agreed to subsidize.

To surprise their parents, Boris and Bob arranged to have their parents' furniture, clothing, kitchenware, and all other belongings shipped and delivered to the apartment. They spent a full day putting the place in some kind of order that they thought would please their parents.

When Ivan and Sophie arrived, Boris and his wife, Janet, and Bob and his wife, Adele, and their two children, Jennifer, twelve, and April, ten, met them at the station. Initially, there was much joy, and Sophie cried when she met her family and saw the new apartment, which was about equidistant from both sons' homes. She cried even more when she saw most of what was in her old home crammed into the small apartment. And so began a new life in a new place for Ivan and Sophie.

Now, months later, the euphoria of being reunited and living in the same city has waned. The first negative experience was when Ivan discovered that he was very intimidated driving in Montreal. The sheer volume of traffic scared him, and he found himself easily confused by the bilingual signs everywhere. Yet driving was important to him; having a car and being able to drive was, for Ivan, an important symbol of his independence. Now he was hardly driving at all.

Both Ivan and Sophie have found getting around the city without the help of their sons to be difficult, if not impossible. They find the city's public transportation intimidating. The subways are frightening, and they feel unsure of themselves on the escalators, in the subway cars, or even in knowing how to get to where they want to go. In short, Ivan and Sophie feel lost and confused by Montreal's size and its very different culture. They miss their friends and the city that for so long was home and that they knew so well.

But worse for them is that they have a strong sense that Boris's and Bob's wives are resentful of the time their husbands spend with their parents. Neither Janet nor Adele call or come to visit very often, and when they do, or when Ivan and Sophie go to their homes for a visit or a meal, there is always a feeling of tension and discomfort. But just as hard to bear for Ivan and Sophie is that their two granddaughters are completely alien and show no interest in or respect for them. When they spend any time at all with Jennifer and April, it's strained and unsatisfying.

After nearly nine months in Montreal, Ivan and Sophie are miserable, lonely, dejected, and depressed. They see their sons less frequently and are certain it's because the wives are exerting pressure on Boris and Bob — which, in fact, is the case.

Meanwhile, Janet and Adele continue to lobby their husbands for more of their time, and for more time with their own parents. It's now become a subtle battle of wills to see whose parents will get what level of attention.

Boris and Bob are confused; they thought they'd done the right thing, for all the right reasons. They're further agitated by the behaviour of their wives, which they'd never anticipated and can't fully understand.

Then, when their parents tell them they would rather return to Red Deer, the brothers are frustrated and angry. In their minds, they've been very responsible and logical, and they can't understand why their parents aren't content and, in fact, grateful. Nor can they understand why their parents don't go out on their own more often and meet people in the Ukrainian community. Both Boris and Bob have taken them to the Ukrainian Orthodox church in Montreal and to a Ukrainian social club, where they thought their parents would find some new friends.

But their parents are adamant about their unhappiness and their desire to move back to Red Deer. Even though their health is slowly deteriorating, Ivan and Sophie are still capable of independent living, and they tell their sons that while they love them dearly, this arrangement isn't working out at all.

THE HEALTH CARE PROFESSIONAL'S POINT OF VIEW

Nothing is as disappointing as disappointment. We often have ideas of what people are like and how we can create situations that will ensure their happiness or at least contentment. But these fantasies are often very different from the actualities of everyday life. That is why everyone is disappointed in the outcome of Boris and Bob's plans for their parents and the reality of Ivan and Sophie's day-to-day lives in Montreal.

Moving is hard for anyone, and a new situation is often fraught with unknown experiences and unanticipated responses. Whether a move is for work, study, or personal obligations, most people adapt out of necessity. And sometimes a move means immediate success — perhaps a better job, a nicer house, new challenges, and often new friends. But when a move happens later in life, it can be much more difficult. Most people's dearest friends are from the earlier years of life, and such bonding is not easily duplicated in later years. The shared memories and reference points for collective reminiscing, such an important part of social activity, is lost as the fabric of friends is disrupted by death or by a move away.

So what happened here with this clearly caring family that might have been averted, and is there any way to salvage the situation?

First of all, a decision to move an older relative must be made with careful thought. A family can rarely be a sufficient substitute for a social network. Families may care for loved ones more in the deepest sense, but they cannot replace the normal social activities of a familiar circle of friends in a long-accustomed environment.

Before considering the move, Boris and Bob should have discussed with their parents what it was that they thought they would need in order to be reasonably satisfied, if not happy, in Montreal. If all the answers were focused on the closeness of the family, everyone might have stepped back and asked, "Is that going to be enough?" Also, some frank discussion with spouses and children should have taken place in order to avoid feelings of hurt or abandonment. A spouse or children can easily feel that their usual family time is lost when so much time and attention shifts to the care of elderly parents.

It might have been worthwhile to try out the arrangement, perhaps giving it a chance with a three- or four-month visit, using a rented apartment or house and not moving everything out right away. This would have given Ivan and Sophie an opportunity to figure out what there is in the new community that might be attractive enough to make the move worthwhile, separate from the anticipated need to be with family as their faculties decline and health becomes compromised.

If, after a prolonged visit, Sophie and Ivan felt that they would likely be isolated, perhaps a permanent move would not have been contemplated. Some families choose to have a number of prolonged visits to provide an opportunity for the parents to explore and make some acquaintances that might form the nucleus of new friendships should a permanent move be undertaken. The sons could not possibly fill the void left by the loss of the network that Ivan and Sophie had in Red Deer. Children are rarely friends with their parents, and the child-parent role is hard to change even in mature years.

For their part, Ivan and Sophie should have had a heart-to-heart talk with each other to understand why they decided to make the move. They needed to understand that while they would be losing some of their present happiness in Red Deer, they would at least be with family and feel secure should something go wrong. There is nothing wrong with that choice, but when they made it, they needed to decide to dedicate themselves to finding ways to make it work, rather than comparing their new situation to what they had before. Such a move could never result in their having the same milieu that existed with their friends in Red Deer. But if they felt that the modest amount of loneliness and lack of social network was worth the investment in the future, then they might have come to terms with the trade-off. Clearly they had the strength during their younger years to make such a choice, but in later years it was less easy to do.

Finally, Boris and Bob need not feel that they failed. They also cannot blame their families for letting their parents down. It would be an extraordinary family that could accept a major shift of attention from their lives to the needs of parents now living in the community without some feeling of resentment. This would be true even when coupled with great filial dedication to care for one's parents and those of one's spouse.

Because things are not working out the family needs to explore the alternatives, the last one being that Ivan and Sophie be allowed to move back to Red Deer, either temporarily or permanently. A frank discussion with everyone in the family, without any blame or suggestion that anyone is at fault, might help clear the air. A counsellor might help the discussion, but one is not necessary for this situation to be fully explored with everyone involved.

Sometimes people imagine the past as being better than the present. Maybe, indeed, life would be better if Ivan and Sophie moved back to Red Deer. But perhaps not. They may not be able to realign themselves with their previous network. They could try moving back for a few months, renting a suitable place that would not require them to move all their belongings again. Or, they could decide as a family that the future was so risky for Ivan and Sophie that everyone is going to have to sacrifice a bit for things to work out.

Ivan and Sophie are going to have to discard their illusion that their life in Montreal is going to be as good as their life in Red Deer. They need to figure out what they can do to make it as good as possible. They clearly had the strength to make difficult moves in the past, and now they have to draw on their strength to do it again. They need to decide to force themselves to join activities or centres that might provide them with a new network of acquaintances and activities, even if they aren't ideal. The attitude with which they undertake that task will go a long way in determining their success. I have seen many of my patients resist joining a club or taking on a volunteer position only to thank me later because of the successful outcome they had when they finally took a chance.

Boris's and Bob's families have to come to some agreement about how they will deal with Ivan and Sophie living nearby. This should include a commitment to spend a reasonable amount of time with them, knowing that in all likelihood things will improve with time if everyone is very caring and supportive in the beginning. It is not too late to salvage the situation.

Boris and Bob should admit to their parents that they made some mistakes moving them to Montreal, but tell them that there is a time to try to turn things around. And they should remind their parents that the reason for the decision to move in the first place was the concern that Ivan or Sophie, or both of them, might need help in the near future because of failing health. Bob and Boris would not be able to provide that help in Red Deer, and Ivan and Sophie could end up quite isolated in that community. Ivan and Sophie should agree to give the move another try for about four months. During this time they could join some social groups and really make an effort to see what might happen if they attempted to meet people and develop a new network of friends.

The agreement might be that if, after four months of everyone trying their best to explore the relationship, build on its strengths, and understand the long-term benefits for the future, things are not better, Ivan and Sophie will move back to Red Deer. If so, Boris and Bob will not have failed, nor will have their families.

In due course the situation may resolve itself, if, for example, Ivan and Sophie need medical care in Red Deer and receive it there, or if they progressively deteriorate so that they cannot look after themselves but find somewhere to stay in that community. Or perhaps after one parent dies, the one who survives will accept that there are no real choices but to rejoin their children in Montreal.

No matter what decision is made, it is important to remember that this experience was not a failure, but merely a human attempt to be a loving family. Plans don't always turn out the way we would like them to, and that is just the way things are, even when those plans are made with the best of intentions.

BREAKING THE MOLD:

The Rebellious Grandmother

Sometimes we make assumptions about our parents that are wrong, and that can lead to negative consequences, as in this case of an elderly woman whose daughter mistakenly decides what her mother would like to do.

THE CHALLENGE

Fatima Campenello is a seventy-four-year-old widow who never mastered English, despite living in Canada for fifty years. She and her husband, Julio, moved to Canada from their native Italy in 1952, the day after her twenty-fifth birthday. On arrival, they landed in Toronto's large Italian community, where for the first few years they lived in a one-bedroom apartment and started life anew.

Julio's cousin, who had come to Toronto several years earlier, already had a relatively good job in a bakery, and he helped Julio and Fatima settle in. While Julio soon landed a job working as a shipping dock hand at the city's food and produce terminal, Fatima found nothing after considerable searching. Eventually, though, she started cleaning homes in the area. She also spent considerable time babysitting for neighbours and even for some of the clients for whom she cleaned. And so cleaning and looking after young children became her full-time work for many years.

In 1964, when Fatima was thirty-seven and Julio forty-two, Fatima became pregnant and gave birth to their only child, Angela. While both were delighted at the arrival of the child, it was a surprise coming fairly late in their lives.

Fatima lavished time and attention on her daughter while still working five days a week cleaning homes and babysitting. If she had to babysit in the evenings, she'd often take Angela along so she could spend time with her daughter and her daughter could play with new friends.

Eventually, the Campenellos moved into a two-bedroom unit of a fourplex, still in Toronto's Italian community. Twice they made the pilgrimage back their old hometown in southern Italy, and over the years a few relatives came to visit them.

Angela thrived in school and revelled in her cultural heritage. She learned to speak fluent Italian and to read and write in the language. Her English was also flawless. She graduated with honours from high school and went on to earn a university degree in psychology with top grades.

Once she finished her schooling, she found a job in a teen counselling centre. In her late twenties, Angela married Frank Combriani, a hardworking chartered accountant whose parents had also emigrated from Italy in the early 1950s. For the first few years of their marriage, Angela and Frank lived in a downtown apartment; later they bought a small house in suburban Scarborough. When Julio retired at age sixty-six, Fatima continued to babysit a few half-days a week. The extra income was welcome and she enjoyed the work. Over the years she had gained a strong reputation for her skill with children. In fact, she was babysitting the children of some of those she had babysat years earlier. In their increasing free time, Julio and Fatima socialized, still staying for the most part in their Italian community.

Four years ago, Julio, who'd complained with increasing frequency about headaches but had refused for the longest time to see a doctor, was diagnosed with a brain tumour. Surgery was determined to be too risky, and his age further compounded the situation. Julio died two years ago.

For a period of time after his death, Fatima continued to live on her own in their small home but found it increasingly difficult to manage. She explored the option of finding another woman to share the house with, but that seemed complicated. She considered moving into a retirement home, but because she was in relatively good health, the notion of being around so many "old people" left her thinking that wasn't such a good idea.

That's when Angela and Frank suggested to her that she move in with them. By this time they had a five-year-old son, Frank Jr., who was about to start kindergarten, but they had a large house that included a small, self-contained apartment in the basement. After much discussion and a lot of thinking, Fatima decided that perhaps it would be a good move. She loved her daughter, and she was very fond of Frank. A month later, she made the move.

Generally, the transition was good. Fatima liked her little room and her privacy, and she also liked spending time with her grandson. She especially liked her time with her daughter and son-in-law because they could speak comfortably in Italian. She would also watch a considerable amount of Italian television programming, and every few weeks Frank or Angela would take her to visit friends in her old neighbourhood.

Then Angela became pregnant again and delivered a healthy, beautiful daughter, Gabriella — which soon became "Gabby." Angela took six months off work to be home with Gabby, and life seemed to be good for all. When it was time for Angela to go back to work, she asked her mother to babysit Gabby, since she was living with them anyway and it was clear she liked spending time with her. Fatima seemed reluctant, but she did agree, and so Angela didn't give it any further thought as she resumed her work life.

As the months passed, both Frank and Angela noticed that Fatima seemed more withdrawn and, as they saw it, depressed. But whenever they asked Fatima if there was a problem or if she felt well, the response was always the same: a firm denial that anything was wrong, end of conversation. Yet neither Frank nor Angela could accept Fatima's protests, as they could see that her day-to-day behaviour was becoming evermore inwardly focused.

Finally, Angela called a nearby geriatric clinic to arrange an assessment and then broke the news to her mother. She told her mother that she was simply worried about her, and disguised her true concern by explaining that, given her age, Fatima needed to be seen by those specializing in the health of the elderly.

Mother and daughter went to the clinic for the appointment. The geriatrician first met with Fatima and Angela together, and Angela explained that her mother seemed increasingly depressed. She shared that her mother was withdrawn and preferred to spend more and more time in her room, whereas just months ago she seemed to really enjoy family interaction and playing with her grandchildren. Fatima did not contradict her daughter's depiction of the situation.

Then the physician started his examination of Fatima alone, during which time he asked her what was going on from her perspective. He noted that he could not find anything physically wrong with her but was concerned about her mood. He told her she seemed down and "blue." Although her English was not perfect, Fatima was able to express herself adequately enough to explain that she didn't want to babysit her new granddaughter. Fatima explained that she'd been looking after people's children and homes for most of her life, and that she was tired of looking after others — whether they were children or adults. She said she loved her grandchildren, but she wanted to enjoy them and not feel like she had to work at it five days a week.

The geriatrician told her that she had to be honest with her daughter about her feelings, but Fatima initially balked, saying she did not want to hurt her daughter, whom she loved very much. The doctor said he would help her explain and that everything would be all right.

When the geriatrician told Angela what Fatima had said, Angela was shocked. She and Frank had assumed that because her mother had spent so much time babysitting over the years that she'd be very comfortable continuing to do so with her own grandchildren. Plus, they trusted Fatima with Gabby and Frank Jr. And, truth be known, the arrangement helped them reduce expenses. But mostly, Angela said, they had believed that her mother would thrive in looking after her grandchildren; this, after all, is what both remembered seeing so much of in their old Italian neighbourhood in their youth.

Angela expressed regret that she had put her mother in this unfair situation and said she wanted to help resolve the situation in any way suitable to Fatima. With this freedom bestowed on her, Fatima generously offered a few days a week to act in her loving grandmotherly role while knowing that she had the other days for herself, to explore and grow in areas that appealed to her.

The Health Care Professional's Point of View

The experience of Fatima, Angela, and Frank is a perfect example of wrong assumptions that may lead to family strife and, in this case, an almost pathological emotional state on the part of one member of the family. Almost any family situation can result in misunderstandings, and if they aren't addressed in an open and honest way, they can lead to family dysfunction and disruptions that last for many years and, if not dealt with, become irreversible.

Sometimes stereotyping of traditional gender-based roles may interfere with a family member's ability to fulfill his or her personal goals and expectations. Many older women recall their childhood experiences when they were directed to choose a career path or personal direction based on assumptions of what was right for a girl. Of course, nowadays that is less common, and most mature women feel they have the right and personal obligation to fulfill their own interests and aspirations. We may forget, however, that our parents may feel the same way, even though they have never had the chance to act that way in the past.

An important key to mature and respectful relationships is open and honest communication. When we feel thwarted or unable to address an important personal issue because of fear of rejection or anger or disappointment, we may turn in to ourselves and develop the kind of symptoms that Fatima manifested, in this case what appeared to be a depressive state.

She felt trapped by the assumptions made by her daughter and her own true devotion to her child and her grandchildren. She was even willing to make the personal sacrifice of not addressing the issue with her daughter, but her deep emotional strife manifested itself in her behaviour. It is fortunate that Angela, being a caring and sensitive daughter, sought to help her mother without realizing the source of her emotional problem.

Fatima did not have the courage or perhaps the practice of expressing her own wishes or needs and accepted the situation rather than disappoint her daughter. This is where a knowledgeable and sensitive physician can play a crucial role in helping to solve a family problem. The trust that most people feel toward their doctor allows the physician to use his or her experience and knowledge to influence the decisions that families make. In this case, giving Fatima the opportunity to express herself privately to the doctor, away from her daughter, was key to figuring out what was going on. All older patients, when visiting a doctor, especially a new one, should have the opportunity to speak to the doctor alone and in confidence, if they are able to do so. Many doctors structure their interview to include all family members during the initial history taking and then examine the patient alone, thereby allowing the person to express his or her own feelings in private. Doctors should try to structure their visits to accommodate this need to speak to the patient privately and confidentially.

Once the issue is recognized it is important to discuss it with everyone involved, and here again the physician can play a role in helping the different players in the situation understand that there is no blame involved but rather a misunderstanding that led to an unfortunate decision. In this case, Angela's response was most crucial. Had she berated her mother for not being a caring parent and grandparent, or made her feel guilty by saying that she had decided to go back to work based on knowing that Fatima would be looking after the infant, Fatima may have changed her mind, acquiesced, and then been resentful for many years to come.

This situation worked out well because of Angela's willingness to be open and respectful and the physician's insight in discerning that there was something wrong that did not fit into the usual picture of clinical depression. The result is likely to be fruitful and satisfying for everyone, with the possibility of Fatima expanding her free days or contracting them, depending on which of her activities gives her the most satisfaction. Or she may continue with the same mix of time, thereby enjoying both her family and her own new achievements and personal growth.

CULTURE CLASH:

Pitting Values against Needs

When hard, pragmatic decisions are required, differing views and values of parents, their children, and those who influence them can lead to new challenges when trying to decide on the right thing to do.

THE CHALLENGE

Moshe and Miriam Greenberg were born in Poland. They were teenagers when they met in Warsaw, and both they and their families became very good friends. When the Nazis invaded their country, Moshe was twenty-one and Miriam had just turned nineteen.

As Poland crumbled under the onslaught of the Germans' massive war machine, both Moshe's and Miriam's families wanted to flee, but by then the options were few and far between. Trapped, as were hundreds of thousands of other Jewish families, they tried to live their lives as normally as possible. However, that didn't last long at all.

For the first year of German occupation, Moshe and Miriam and their families remained in their homes, although day by day their world kept deteriorating until it was shattered completely when the Nazis announced they would be "moved." That move, of course, was to a concentration camp. Two days before they were herded into trucks, Moshe and Miriam were married in a secret ceremony because they wanted to be together forever — whatever "forever" would come to mean for them.

What followed was almost five years of unimaginable personal terror and horror for each of them. They watched in anguish and anger as family members and friends died before their eyes or simply vanished, never to be seen again. Sometimes, Moshe and Miriam didn't know for weeks on end whether the other was even alive. But because they were young and in good health at the outset, and because they both had a fierce will to live, at war's end both were still alive — barely. It was weeks after their camp had been liberated that Moshe and Miriam were reunited, both of them mentally and physically scarred.

They slowly recovered their health, and once the emotional pain had subsided to a manageable level, Moshe and Miriam knew they had to get on with rebuilding their world, which was now empty of all their families and most of their friends. Fortunately, Moshe had a cousin who lived in Montreal who sponsored them to come to Canada.

Moshe and Miriam adjusted to their new world with remarkable agility. Thanks to some helping hands and their own sense of drive and purpose, the young couple soon had good entry-level jobs: Moshe learned the tool and die business while Miriam, who had a special skill with numbers, learned to be a bookkeeper in a small textile company.

They worked hard, saved money as they could, and forged ahead. In 1952 they bought a small house on the outskirts of the city, and a year later Miriam gave birth to their first child, a son they named Seth. Two years later she had another son, Isaac. Helen was born eighteen months later.

As the years moved on, the Greenberg family remained very close-knit. Moshe and Miriam were very traditional in their religious beliefs and practices, and carefully and thoughtfully observed all the Jewish holidays. Moshe took his sons to synagogue every Friday night and often talked to them about the importance of their heritage and the huge pains inflicted on their family and their people during the course of history, and especially during the past world war.

Eventually, Moshe and Miriam's children reached adulthood and each went off in search of his or her own destiny. Seth became a chartered accountant and landed a good job with a Toronto-based firm specializing in the lucrative field of forensic accounting. Isaac, who had always loved music and was an accomplished pianist, studied business in university and ended up managing a number of rock groups, bands, and singers. Helen studied physiotherapy and started a small but successful clinic with three partners that grew into a real going concern.

As the children moved ahead with their own lives, Moshe noted that Seth, Isaac, and Helen and their families spent less and less time with their parents, and they seemed to drift away from the strong religious grounding he and Miriam had instilled.

Several years ago, Moshe and Miriam moved into a retirement home that had an adjacent long-term nursing facility. They continued to live fairly independently, with daily support services. Their three children and their spouses and grandchildren visited regularly and phoned often to check on them and discuss their needs.

Now, Moshe is eighty-two years old. His health has been steadily failing over the past five years. First, he was diagnosed as a diabetic. A year later, he suffered a mild heart attack that left him weakened and tentative because he was afraid of another, more severe, attack. But instead of another heart attack, Moshe suffered a stroke, and then another. Since his second stroke, Moshe has been unable to speak or move his left arm or leg. He's lost control of his bowels and is having a very difficult time chewing his food. Late last year, Moshe was trans-ferred to the long-term nursing facility, while Miriam moved to a smaller apartment in the retirement home.

At eighty, Miriam is still vigorous and mentally alert. She visits her husband at least twice a day and sometimes sits with him for several hours at a time.

Seth, Isaac, and Helen have discussed their father's health, acknowledging that he is on a course of steady deterioration. They have talked with their mother about the future, urging her to consider allowing him to pass on if there are any further complications.

Miriam was very upset about her children's suggestion and turned to her rabbi for advice. Rabbi Rubinfeld was very clear and firm in his counsel to her: the sanctity of life is more important than any other factor, he told her. He said that was true in Judaism and every other religion, and that no matter what, every effort must always be made — with no exceptions — to keep any living being alive. Miriam accepted his wisdom totally and told her children how she felt.

What her children saw, though, was a father who was a shell of the man they knew and whose life was barely livable. But their mother made it clear that she was in charge of the situation, and that as long as she was of sound mind her first priority was to keep her husband alive. Besides, she told them, there were new medicines and treatments coming on the market almost every day, and she knew that people in their father's condition did improve sometimes, so that couldn't be ruled out, either.

In what they thought might be a good step to take, Seth, Isaac, and Helen decided that Seth should meet with Rabbi Rubinfeld and ask for his support. Seth explained to the rabbi that he and his brother and sister were worried about their father's quality of life, and he asked the rabbi to help prepare their mother for a difficult decision that was bound to have to be made sometime. The rabbi, however, was steadfast and told Seth that he couldn't help, given his own strong convictions.

Meanwhile, Moshe contracted pneumonia and required treatment with antibiotics and oxygen, but he recovered. But it was clear to the physicians and nurses that he contracted pneumonia because of the difficulty he has swallowing. They felt that he would need a feeding tube to provide nourishment and fluids to maintain him and to reduce the risk of further episodes of pneumonia. The doctor at the nursing home asked Miriam what she would like to do. He said they could try feeding him again, but that if he developed another bout of pneumonia he could die from it. On the other hand, the feeding tube had some risks, although for the most part it was a fairly safe procedure.

The doctor also explained the situation to Seth when he came to check on his father. Seth called his sister and brother to tell them about the choice they had to make. One of the nurses caring for Moshe indicated to Seth in private that she thought it would be cruel to prolong their father's suffering by putting in a tube and that she could never understand families who made that decision. On a different occasion two nurses spoke to Helen and said that Miriam was so devoted that even with a tube her father could still have some meaningful and comfortable life ahead of him.

The three siblings then arranged to visit their mother, and they pleaded with her to let events take their course without putting in a feeding tube, which they felt would just prolong their father's suffering. Only Helen was ambivalent about not feeding her father — not so much for religious reasons, but because of the idea of "starving" him, especially with her knowledge of the symbolic meaning of food for her parents because of the Holocaust experience. Seth and Isaac told their mother that while they loved their father, watching him like this was very painful for them and they wondered if he would have wanted a feeding tube had he been able to make such a decision himself. They felt he would not.

Miriam was furious. She told Seth and Isaac that she felt they were betraying their father and their faith. She appealed to Helen for support. She said that since she was the decision-maker she simply wouldn't talk about it any more because she believed Moshe, as an observant Jew, would want to follow Rabbi Rubinfeld's advice. She reminded them of the terrible ordeal she and Moshe had experienced so many years ago and said that was evidence that one should never, ever give up on living.

Now, there is a high level of tension between Seth, Isaac, and their mother, with Helen not quite sure if her mother is right in making this decision. They would like the rabbi to be more "realistic" in the advice he is giving to their mother.

THE HEALTH CARE PROFESSIONAL'S POINT OF VIEW

Conflicts over cultural, ethnic, and religious perspectives are common in any multicultural society. In the health care profession, we usually think of the conflict as being one in which a patient and family have their own peculiar perspective which is not understood or shared by the health care team, thereby leading to unnecessary conflicts. In fact, many health care organizations and health care professionals seek ways to get advice about and assistance with cultures they do not fully understand.

There are many cases in which the health care staff, because of a failure to understand and appreciate the underlying values and beliefs that determine a family's decision, end up in situations of terrible conflict. There are even cases that have made their way through the court system because, for example, a family's belief in the sanctity of life persuaded them to demand that the patient be kept on a respirator following a severe motor vehicle accident, even though the health care team felt that the there was no chance of a good recovery and that it was a waste to continue with intensive care treatments. In other cases, some health care team members might be so intent on allowing the patient to have the final say that they fail to recognize and appreciate that in a particular culture it is the accepted practice for the eldest son to make a decision and protect the parent from the pain associated with such a step.

All religious, cultural, and ethnic groups have beliefs and rituals with special meaning and importance to those who follow the tenets of the particular group involved. It is important for health care providers to understand where decisions come from so that they can best support the decision-makers.

In this particular case, the problem appears to be an estrangement of underlying values between Miriam and at least two of her children, coupled with different health care team members providing conflicting advice to family members. It is often the case that different generations with different life experiences have incongruent value systems when facing difficult end-of-life situations. As for the staff, they should not be providing advice based on their own personal values to a family in turmoil. Rather, they should limit their advice to the factual level of whether feeding tubes could safely provide nourishment to Moshe and decrease the risk of aspiration pneumonia.

What is the best way to support this family and do everything possible to help them through a difficult period so that after Moshe dies they will still be a loving and caring family?

First of all, the children have to accept that their mother is the rightful surrogate decision-maker, whether they agree with her values or not, and that she appears to be acting in a way that is consistent with Moshe's religious beliefs. From their past actions, it is clear that Miriam and Moshe take pride in their Judaism and have expressed a commitment to follow its tenets. For most observant Jews, this would mean that when there is a difficult situation and a rabbi's advice is sought, that advice must be followed.

For Miriam, the concept of sanctity of life is very important, and its importance was emphasized to her by the rabbi she consulted. He also would have told her that providing food is an obligation except when doing so itself causes harm, and so giving Moshe a feeding tube would be an extension of that obligation to feed.

If Moshe was not likely to survive the pneumonia and was in fact dying, the rabbi might very well have given different advice to Miriam. For most religious Jews, the obligations concerning the care of a dying person are different; comfort becomes paramount, so a feeding tube might not be inserted.

For Miriam, it is clear that the religious rules and obligations are important to her husband, as they are to her. She would likely take great comfort after Moshe dies knowing that she assured his care was in the religious tradition of Judaism, even if the outcome was not what she wanted. If, on the other hand, she were to ignore what she believed his wishes would be, she would likely carry the guilt with her for the rest of her life and blame herself for not doing the right thing. The children, who are no longer committed to Jewish tradition and law (known as Halacha), may fail to appreciate that certain rules exist that may not make sense to them in a secular world. Similar value systems are shared by Muslims and many of the Catholic faith. On the other hand, people from Southeast Asia may approach the same situation differently from someone from South America and still differently from someone from the Caribbean.

Seth and Isaac may have difficulty understanding why Miriam is so intent on trying to keep their father alive when he appears to have such a poor quality of life. Helen appears to be in a better position to support her mother's wishes, whatever they may be, and that will be very important for Miriam as she struggles through this difficult period. It is terrible to feel alone when making difficult decisions, and the support of a parent's children is often key to his or her ability to survive emotionally during trying situations.

It might be worthwhile for Seth and Isaac, if they have forgotten the basic tenets of Judaism when it comes to decisions such as these, to meet with the rabbi privately for an explanation of the basis of the decision. Even if they long ago abandoned their own Jewish religious beliefs, they are likely able to project sufficiently to understand the basic underpinnings of the faith and how it affects decisions. If they could successfully bring themselves to see the situation from their mother's perspective, they could likely be a great support to her. Even if in their own hearts Seth and Isaac disagree with the decision, if they can accept that it is consistent with their parents' belief system and embrace it and its possible consequences (i.e., Moshe being kept alive for a period of time with a feeding tube in place), it would go a long way to restoring family peace.

For families in which the value-based ties have been splintered, it is important that the children step back a bit and try to imagine the values of their parents. By doing this, they should be able to understand the importance of following through in the practice of the religion or culture that they hold. Many people who appear to have abandoned their religion during their adult years find comfort in the traditions and practices as they approach death. There is nothing inconsistent or hypocritical in this shift, and everything should be done to support people who need to revert to previously held beliefs, even those they may have ignored for years, if that is what makes them comfortable during their remaining days.

Seth, Isaac, and Helen should try to find a way to gather around Miriam and tell her that whatever decision she makes is the right one and that they understand the Judaic reasons for the decision and support her in that difficult choice.

If Moshe lives for many months, even if he does not improve at all, they must not waver in their support of her decision. If, on the other hand, a tube is inserted and Moshe succumbs, they can feel comfort in the fact that they supported their mother's decision to do the right thing according to Judaism. That support will give her comfort for the days, months, and years ahead when she thinks about what transpired during those terrible days of Moshe's last illness.

SUBSTANCE ABUSE:

Drinking All Day Keeps Reality Away

Parents who are unwilling or unable to cope with their lives sometimes resort to excessive drinking or taking too many medications. It is especially dangerous if drugs and alcohol are mixed, which can lead to dire consequences and to huge concerns for the children.

THE CHALLENGE

Gilles Ducet is a seventy-eight-year-old widower who lives in a small two-bedroom home in Trois Rivières, Quebec. Gilles was a construction worker from the time he left school when he was seventeen until he retired at age sixty-six. Over the years, Gilles worked hard; he was physically strong because of the type of work he did. He always liked to have a few beers with his buddies at the end of the day, followed by several shots of whiskey in the evenings after dinner. When Gilles retired, he kept drinking but began putting on weight because he wasn't nearly as physically active.

His wife, Hélène, died six years ago of cancer. They were very close and her death was a terrible blow for Gilles. He retreated into his house, and further into himself, for several years. And he drank more, although he denied it to his twin fifty-two-year-old daughters, Eva and Estelle.

Two years ago, Gilles was in a minor car accident late one night and was charged with impaired driving. His licence was suspended, and although he can now reapply for a licence, he has not done so. The fact is that Gilles rarely leaves his house since the accident; the most he does outdoors is mow his small lawn in the summer and sweep the snow if it's not too deep during the long winter months.

Estelle, who is divorced and lives alone, works as a real estate broker in Trois Rivières. She visits her father once a week for an hour or two, but because she often finds him tipsy, argumentative, and moody, she rarely enjoys the visits.

Eva lives in Montreal with her second husband; they have no children and are financially secure, which in their case means they often enjoy travelling to distant destinations for several weeks at a time. Eva visits her father about once a month and calls weekly, although, like her sister, she doesn't derive much pleasure or satisfaction from the encounters.

About a year ago, Gilles met and became friends with Claudia, a widow who is ten years younger than Gilles and lives in a nearby apartment building. Claudia now spends most of her time with Gilles at his home.

In comparing notes, Estelle and Eva agree that Claudia seems to tolerate their father's drinking. In fact, they believe Gilles gives Claudia money to buy his beer and whiskey. They also find that Claudia is not particularly open or friendly with either of them, and she usually defends Gilles in any discussion about his lifestyle or drinking. As worrisome to the daughters, they believe that their father is lavishing gifts on Claudia, and that Claudia is under the misguided impression that, despite his meagre lifestyle, Gilles has a lot of money.

Both Estelle and Eva have noticed over the past few months that their father's tolerance for whiskey has declined, but not his consumption. This, of course, results in his being inebriated most of the time. And recently Estelle discovered that her father is also taking tranquilizers prescribed by his doctor.

Although she didn't like doing it, Estelle called the doctor to ask him about the tranquilizers and whether he knew about Gilles's drinking. The doctor acknowledged that he knew Gilles was an occasional drinker but not that he drank as much as Estelle claimed. The doctor also confided that he gave Gilles the prescription because at his last visit Gilles said he was still very depressed about Hélène's death and about his own deteriorating condition. It was clear to Estelle from this conversation that Gilles has never talked to his doctor about his drinking and that the doctor hasn't picked up on the problem.

Estelle then called Eva, and the two of them went to visit their father. They confronted him about the drinking, but he denied that he drank too much and was very defensive. They also told him that they were worried about what to them appeared to be memory lapses and poor judgment during recent visits and telephone calls, and they wondered if mixing the liquor with the tranquilizers was wreaking havoc on his mind and body. If anything, they told their father, he seemed more depressed than ever.

Gilles was adamant in his rebuttal of his daughters' allegations and dismissed their concerns. He got quite angry and told them that his life was much better now that Claudia was part of it, how she looked after him with much more care and attention than his own daughters, and how much that meant to him. Then he told them that he'd asked Claudia to move in with him. They would both benefit, their father explained, because Gilles would always have someone around, and Claudia would be able to save the money she paid for her apartment. It was at this point in their heated exchange that Claudia arrived, and a strained, polite, and inconsequential conversation followed before Estelle and Eva left.

The sisters both went home. Later that night they had a long telephone debate about what to do and how to do it. They agreed that most worrisome for them was Claudia's move into the house with their father. Not only didn't they particularly like or trust Claudia, but more importantly they felt certain the woman would continue to supply their father with all the beer and whiskey he wanted. In addition, they feared Claudia had a self-serving agenda: to save her own money and live off Gilles's limited savings.

The more Eva and Estelle talked, the more other fears surfaced, like the thought that Claudia would somehow manipulate their father into assigning ownership of the house to her, or talk him into giving her power of attorney and then having him institutionalized, selling the house, and walking away with what was left of his modest savings. They also worried about their father's failing health and mental capacity, but they didn't know what to do next because they weren't sure Gilles's doctor was paying close enough attention to the real needs of his patient.

The Health Care Professional's Point of View

This is a difficult situation for Gilles's daughters. They should have many concerns, the first being the psychological and physical well-being of their father.

Gilles is on a path to the almost certain severe consequences that result from consuming excessive alcohol combined with tranquilizers. The risk is twofold: first is the negative effect of alcohol on his neurological function and the potentially serious damage to other organs such as his liver, and second is the effect of his depression on his health. Alcohol and tranquilizers aggravate depression, and if no intervention takes place, Gilles will be at risk for doing something serious such as committing suicide.

Older men have a very high suicide rate, and when they decide on the act they often succeed, using rather violent methods such as hanging or guns. If Gilles is indeed depressed over his wife's death, he might benefit from medical treatment of a combination of antidepressant medication coupled with counselling or psychotherapy.

Another confounding aspect to this situation is the role of Claudia. The children may be suspicious of her intentions, but she may, in fact, have true affection for Gilles with no ulterior motives. Whatever the situation, the daughters will likely require her co-operation in their attempt to help their father. If they find that she is an obstacle to his well-being, the situation is more complex and may require some legal action to protect their father.

Assuming that Claudia cares for Gilles but does not realize the risks of his drinking and use of tranquilizers, Estelle and Eva must discuss the situation with her. They will need Claudia's assistance to achieve their goals of getting Gilles to stop drinking and taking tranquilizers, and of getting proper treatment for his depression. They will also need the assistance of Gilles's family physician, with whom they should have a meeting.

The sequence of meetings depends on whether Claudia is in agreement with them about Gilles's condition or is part of the problem. If Claudia proves to be an ally, she might join them when they meet with the doctor. Or she might prefer to defer to the daughters to outline the situation to the doctor and confirm that she is willing to co-operate in any fashion required to assist Gilles, for whom she cares a lot.

At the meeting with the doctor, the daughters must impress upon him that they are observing serious changes in their father's mood and cognitive function. They must use words and examples that describe sufficiently their observations so that the doctor can understand that Gilles is doing his best to hide the extent of his drinking and is not adequately expressing the degree of his depression. If the physician agrees to assist Estelle and Eva, an appointment should be made for Gilles to see the doctor. This can be arranged either by the daughters or at the initiation of the doctor.

The daughters should explain to Gilles that they have concerns about his drinking and that they really believe a visit to the doctor would be helpful. If he refuses, the doctor might be able to assist by calling Gilles and asking him to visit to make sure that he is all right. Subterfuge in such situations does not usually work because the whole process should be based on trust, and if Gilles begins not to trust his daughters' devotion to him, it will be very hard to resolve this complex situation.

If Gilles agrees to visit his physician, and if Claudia agrees with and supports the goal of decreasing Gilles's alcohol consumption, then

Claudia should accompany the daughters on the visit. Then, together, they can express their love and devotion to Gilles and their desire to help him.

The physician can be extremely helpful in how he approaches Gilles's drinking problem. It is well known that people who abuse alcohol and other drugs that effect mood usually deny their problem. An approach by the physician that is non-judgmental but that rather focuses on the effects on Gilles's mental function is likely to have the best impact. People like Gilles are more likely to listen to a straightforward explanation that continuous exposure of the brain to alcohol can lead to a condition of dementia similar to Alzheimer's disease. Few people are willing to risk the loss of their cognitive function when the implications are laid out (e.g., loss of independence, loss of memory and judgment, inability to perform simple tasks such as dressing and going to the toilet). A discussion about the negative effect on sexual function may also be effective. Gilles may already be aware of this phenomenon but not realize the connection to alcohol use. This discussion should include the potential benefits of using a proper combined therapy for depression with antidepressant medication and counselling.

One visit to the doctor may not be sufficient. The physician should be willing to initiate a process by which to assist Gilles in the very challenging process of recognizing that there is a problem and then taking the steps to address it. The physician may suggest counselling from a social worker or psychologist if there is someone with that expertise available. There may be a special program in the community available for people dealing with substance abuse (the term often used for excessive use of alcohol and medications that effect the brain's function). If so, the physician may recommend that Gilles should access such services.

The most important part of the process is a commitment to help Gilles even if he does not follow through exactly as everyone would like. Sometimes an agreement to cut back gradually on the amount of alcohol consumed is a reasonable first step. This type of arrangement is important to consider because alcohol abusers usually can't imagine completely discontinuing their drinking. Also, when alcohol consumption is suddenly discontinued there is a potential danger of seizures occurring, which can be very frightening and sometimes cause serious injury. So a gradual approach with the support of everyone who cares for Gilles is necessary to achieve the goal.

If things go well, Gilles will gradually decrease his alcohol intake and the tranquilizers will be discontinued. At some point a decision will likely be made to undertake treatment with antidepressants. It is preferable to discontinue using alcohol before starting these drugs, but sometimes, if small doses are started and the results carefully monitored, antidepressants can be introduced while alcohol intake is reduced. Sometimes antidepressant therapy improves the patient's mental state so that the commitment to stop drinking becomes stronger and is more readily implemented.

If these steps are followed through, there is a good chance that Gilles can cease his alcohol abuse and respond properly to antidepressant therapy. He can then have a full relationship with his daughters and, if it proves appropriate, with Claudia.

If the situation proves to be more difficult — with Gilles denying there is a problem and Claudia ignoring the concerns of his daughters — the approach is more complex and may require legal intervention. If Claudia is acting in a malicious manner and taking advantage of Gilles, then Eva and Estelle are faced with finding a way to have her influence on Gilles diminished or removed altogether. This will not be easy and may result in Gilles and his daughters becoming alienated. If Eva and Estelle are convinced that no alternative is possible, they may have to pursue a legally based course of action. If this is necessary, Gilles may not be amenable to the course of action that is best for him in terms of his alcohol use.

The last option for Estelle and Eva is to let things go and not do anything until some crisis occurs, which may allow them to intervene without causing an affront to Gilles. Such a crisis might be a severe medical consequence of his drinking, such as bleeding from his stomach, a seizure, or severe loss of mental competence that forces decision-making upon the daughters. This is not the way anyone would want the situation resolved, but it may be the only viable option to avoid severe alienation and disruption of the family's fabric and integrity.

SEXUALITY, ROMANCE, AND THE FAMILY:

When Children Worry about Their Parents

What do you do when your elderly mother or father becomes romantically involved at a stage of life in which you think such relationships are no longer appropriate?

THE CHALLENGE

It wasn't easy for Sandra and Denise. On one of their recent visits to the nursing home they were told that their eighty-seven-year-old mother, Margaret, experiencing moderate Alzheimer's dementia, was becoming romantically involved with Louis, a gentleman on the same unit. Sandra and Denise had been feeling quite comfortable during the past year or so since Margaret had moved into the home, as they saw that rather than appearing quite lonely — which was the case when she was living at home, even with all kinds of community supports — she seemed quite happy in her new environment. They had heard from the staff that she was attending arts and crafts activities and social events and had perked up since her admission, even though her memory was still quite poor.

Both the head nurse and social worker told Margaret's daughters that Margaret was showing signs of becoming quite attached to Louis, who had moved into the home about five months ago and had a mild degree of cognitive impairment. The social worker, for reasons of confidentiality, could not reveal to the daughters that Louis had been admitted because he had sustained a stroke from which he made a good recovery. He had been living more and more in isolation, and his family felt that it wasn't safe for him to be at home anymore, and the nursing home seemed to be the best option. He required, in fact, relatively little nursing care, and participated in all the creative and social activities of the nursing home in general and his unit in particular. One of his favourite activities was dancing, and he started to attend the weekly social event that had dancing, to which Margaret often went. They had started dancing together and were already recognized as very good dance partners.

The two sisters heard from the unit staff that Margaret and Louis were spending more and more time together, and that their relationship seemed to be taking on a romantic flavour.

Louis's two sons, Ralph and Phillip, and his daughter, Brenda, were also aware of the growing relationship but didn't seem to be upset by it. They'd mentioned that following their mother's death four years previously, Louis had a female companion for a while, but after that faded he expressed loneliness, and then the decision was made to move him into the nursing home. They see the new relationship with Margaret as having a very positive effect on their father and heard that the staff thought the same about the effect on her. The three children indicated that they'd be happy to meet with Margaret's children, but Sandra and Denise have rejected that offer. Since they visit at different times because of work schedules, they haven't yet bumped into each other even informally. But it's just a matter of time before that happens, and the staff are concerned how they may interact with each other if a formal meeting to discuss the issue is not arranged.

The social worker and one of the senior nurses explained to Denise and Sandra that they have spoken to Margaret about her relationship to Louis and she seems to be able to express her feelings and enjoyment of their romantic relationship. If anything, they say that she likes to talk about it and at times expresses very acceptable insights into the relationship such as, "He makes me laugh," "He makes me feel good," "He reminds of my days with my late husband, Morris, and the fun we used to have," and "I feel like a young girl again." Sandra and Denise discount such comments as being irrelevant to the discussion and revert back to the diagnosis of Alzheimer's disease and their understanding of her incapacity for decision-making.

Sandra and Denise are concerned about what the relationship might lead to, as they have observed their mother acting very affectionately with Louis and believe that she might end up in a sexual rather than just a romantic relationship. In fact, they asked for a formal meeting with the social worker and head nurse. "You have to stop this relationship from going any further. Our mother is not able to understand what is happening to her and she could end up in a difficult position if we do not protect her," they said at the meeting.

"It's not really possible to stop them unless you were to remove her from the unit, or if Louis is transferred, but his children are very happy with where he is," the social worker explained.

Sandra replied, "We are very happy with the unit as well, and until this happened we'd never have thought of moving her. She was here first, so we don't understand why he can't be moved so that our mother is protected."

The staff suggested that maybe further discussions should take place with the facility's ethicist in attendance. There were, according to staff observations, many issues involved for which an ethics perspective might be worthwhile. One of the concerns they discussed among themselves was what would happen if the relationship were allowed to progress: Where could Margaret and Louis go for privacy, since the unit had only double rooms and each of them had a roommate? Also, the structure of the unit didn't facilitate privacy in general, and staff members expressed concern that should the relationship become overtly sexual, it might disturb other residents of the floor or lead to discomfort among other residents and for Margaret and Louis.

The Health Care Professional's Point of View

Sandra and Denise's concern about their mother is understandable. But before they take it upon themselves to force the nursing home to try to separate their mother from Louis, they should really step back a bit and look at the situation through their mother's eyes.

Margaret was always a very warm and affectionate woman, they both admit. She adored their father, and after his death often talked about how lonely she was. She was an attractive woman, and her daughters wondered for the first few years after he died if she might connect with another man, especially at the senior's club or the bridge group she belonged to where there were some eligible men. But she never mentioned that she had any interest.

There was the neighbour who seemed to be interested in her, but Margaret told her daughters that he was "just being a good and helpful neighbour," and then he connected with a woman a good deal younger, and that stopped any musings about a possible relationship. When she started becoming forgetful, she would sometimes appear to lose some of her natural inhibitions and become a bit flirtatious with men, but they did not take it seriously and believed it was just part of her charm, which endeared her to everyone.

But now they are concerned. Although Sandra and Denise admit that she seems very happy and acknowledge intellectually to the social worker that the romantic relationship might be responsible for that sense of well-being, they cannot accept that it could lead to physical sexuality. Even though they consider themselves liberal when it comes to sexuality, the sisters exclude their mother's case from their views, since because of her Alzheimer's disease they do not believe that she really knows what she is doing. They have tried to give her the opportunity to be involved in many decisions about herself, such as choosing which furniture she has in her room and the clothes that she has recently bought and whether or not she wants new glasses, but both Sandra and Denise are adamant that a romantic, and possibly a sexual, relationship is beyond Margaret's mental capabilities.

The social worker asked them again if they would discuss the situation with Ralph, Philip, and Brenda, but the daughters made it clear that the issue is too sensitive for them and that they never discussed sexuality with their mother even during their younger adult years. They admit that they would not even know how to broach the subject without being excessively embarrassed.

One of the problems that children of those suffering from Alzheimer's disease often encounter is determining how much decision-making they can leave up to their parent. Years ago it was believed that a person with Alzheimer's dementia who was deemed incompetent could not be left to make any personal decisions. During the past decade or more, that view has changed considerably.

It is now believed, and clinical practice supports the premise, that competency (often called "capacity") for making decisions relates to the nature of the task under consideration. Therefore, there has been a move to engage and permit many more personal decisions to be made by individuals with Alzheimer's disease, including some of a serious nature related to health care. Some Alzheimer-afflicted individuals appear to be able to accept or refuse serious medical treatments, or to accept or refuse the need to move into a nursing home. Often, they can decide which family member they would like to make decisions for them should they not be able to do so at some future date. The issue of romance and sexuality very well may be an area where those with mild dementia are able to make reasonable and appropriate choices, and depriving them of this option would undermine the important principle of respecting their decision-making and personal dignity.

We know that even when there is no problem with memory or cognition, families may find it difficult when an elderly single parent develops a romantic relationship. There are all kinds of reasons for such feelings, including guilt for the deceased parent, concerns about what other family members and friends might think, and sometimes concerns about money and property should the relationship result in marriage and what is perceived as an interloper enters into the family structure. Not every child is able to look beyond these issues and focus on the well-being and apparent happiness of a parent, just as parents often try to protect their children when they think they are not in a good relationship. Many of us have had such an experience and use it as the basis of our response to a new stage in the romantic situation of a parent, even a well one.

With concerns about dementia, and perhaps the fear of exploitation and possible harm, it is understandable that Sandra and Denise are reacting the way they are toward Louis and the nursing home, which they feel may be complicit in the development of this romance by not impeding its further development. They fault the nursing home for not telling them sooner or trying to separate Margaret and Louis at social events. They even think the nursing home should have told Louis's children that he would have to be moved to another floor, although they realize that he has just as much a right to stay on his current floor and that his children are very content with where he lives and the fact that he has found a female companion who seems to make him happy.

As for the nursing home staff: they are of two minds. Some who are very sensitive to the need for interpersonal relationships among their residents think that what is happening between Margaret and Louis is a very nice development. The feel that both have the mental capacity to be involved with each other and that no one is being exploited. They have witnessed the good feeling between the two of them and know of previous situations where such relationships have developed and have been very positive. Staff members are even trying to figure out how they could provide Louis and Margaret with adequate privacy should their relationship become sexual, so that other residents of the floor and staff members are not embarrassed. They know that some organizations have privacy rooms for this very purpose and wonder if the administration should be asked to make some renovations to the rather large day room so that a small privacy suite could be built for Margaret and Louis and any other couple that may want to be alone together from time to time.

Other members of the staff are mortified. For personal and what they perceive to be ethical reasons, they think the nursing home should take steps to stop further development of the situation, "before it goes too far." They support Sandra and Denise in their concerns and discount the arguments made by the social worker to respect the relationship and by Philip, Brenda, and Ralph, who are happy that their father has become involved in such a way.

Sandra and Denise must consider the repercussions if they act forcibly to end the relationship between their mother and Louis. They cannot force the nursing home to move Louis from the floor to another unit against his will and for no clinical reason, and they know that his children would not agree to it. They do not want to move their mother if they can help it, because they acknowledge that she is flourishing on the unit and that the staff really like her. They would not consider moving her to another facility for the same reason, and because they recall Margaret's reluctance to move into the facility in the first place. The sisters believe a move to another facility might be devastating for their mother.

They want the best for their mother, but they also want to protect her. They may have to go along with the development of the relationship and try to assess whether it is doing more good than harm. Although this might not be easy for them, it is probably the best thing they can do to protect Margaret's dignity while trying to look after her best interests. In addition, rather than maintaining what has become a somewhat adversarial relationship with Brenda, Philip, and Ralph, they should try to engage them in a way that together they can look at what is happening to their respective parent and agree to common goals and measurements to assure themselves that the relationship is providing more good than harm for both parties. This way, should interventions be necessary, they can be carried out in a co-operative rather than an adversarial way.

Since it is likely that everyone wants the same outcome — the well-being of their parent — each family can agree to respect and support each other in this common goal. Such an arrangement would also make it easier for the staff of the nursing home to assess and respond to this budding romance without fear of alienating one family while pleasing the other. This way, everyone involved can deal with the situation in a manner that above all maintains love, respect, and dignity.

TAPPING THE HUMAN SPIRIT:

It's Never Too Late to Create

An elderly parent is losing a sense of purpose, having no driving ambition and few interests. The challenge is to stimulate and invigorate that parent so there will be a regained sense of discovery and satisfaction.

THE CHALLENGE

Lisa called the clinic secretary again.

"I'm really worried about my father. He's begun to say that life is not worth living again, which he hasn't done for more than a year," she reported. The secretary said she would try to arrange for someone to speak to Sam, Lisa's father, an eighty-six-year-old retired family doctor who's been an occasional patient of the geriatric clinic for more than five years.

There already was an appointment scheduled to see Sam in three weeks as a follow-up to a previous appointment two months ago. Since he moved into a retirement home, Lisa reported, Sam's mood has become much more subdued, and, in fact, more passive in general.

An appointment was made with the outreach psychiatry team while the staff at the retirement home was asked to make sure that Sam was managing and safe, given his negative attitude. Over the ensuing few days, a social worker from the outreach team spoke with Sam and Lisa, as well as the nursing director of the home, who was able to discuss the issues with Sam. It appeared that although he was very sad, there was no indication that Sam was experiencing a major depression at a level that would endanger him. Sam told the nursing director that he was looking forward to the appointment, because he had "lots to talk about."

Arriving for the appointment, Sam, as usual, was very well dressed and looked quite well, according to the secretary who signed him in on his arrival at the geriatric clinic. The medical resident, who talked with him as part of the educational experience with the consultant geriatrician, saw Sam first. "He expresses some despair over his life and that he has nothing much to do, which seems to have been exaggerated since he moved into the home, with all of the 'old folks,'" noted the resident in his report. The resident added, "He continues to eat and sleeps pretty well, and he takes his medications as prescribed for his high blood pressure and diabetes and high cholesterol, and the last laboratory results that were sent to us were quite good."

The geriatrician and the medical resident then met with Sam. Sam had come without his daughter, as was his usual habit — he liked the privacy of the interactions but agreed that the geriatrician could speak to his daughter about the visit if she called, which he expected she would do; he knew that she often worried about him. He also admitted that he was in the habit of expressing his feelings to her. Sam acknowledged that sometimes it might worry her, but he also knew that if she were involved she would help get things done.

He had agreed to move into the retirement home, partially at her prodding, because Sam recognized that he could no longer manage in the house that he had lived in alone since his wife's death eight years ago. Although he felt he could manage in his home, it was becoming clear that he needed lots of help; he no longer drove and was becoming dependant on Lisa for all kinds of ordinary activities and admitted that he was also becoming very lonely.

Sam began to explain how he felt to the geriatrician and the medical resident. "Since I moved into the home, I feel that this must be the last stage," he said. "I've lost my independence and the place is full of 'old' people, at least people who are more needy than I am. But in the last two weeks, since I received all those calls, I've started looking at what I might do at the home to make things a bit better. I feel a bit bad that Dr. Able, who was my psychologist and friend for many years, has moved away so I don't really have the kind of support that I really needed during the past few months with the move and everything else that happened to me."

The geriatrician and medical resident reviewed the medical issues and felt that everything was quite well controlled and the medications were being taken properly. Previous attempts to control his mood with antidepressants hadn't been successful mainly because of side effects, and it was felt that the present situation was not a manifestation of a true and deep depressive illness, but rather an existential feeling of worthlessness and lack of meaning, which could be put into perspective considering his past professional life and his gradual losses, culminating in the move into the retirement home, which Sam saw as the end, with little to look forward to, especially with evidence of aging all around him.

It was agreed that the geriatrician and medical resident would explore options with Sam when they went in to visit him together.

The Health Care Professional's Point of View

It is fairly common for older people to feel a loss of meaningfulness and experience various physical illnesses as they age, and in response they do not see any real positive aspect of their future lives. Their reaction depends a great deal on personality and previous experiences and how they have dealt with the many losses of life and the challenges of interpersonal relationships in the past. It seems that men who have been focused during their adult years primarily on their work or profession often suffer the greatest sense of loss when they can no longer participate in those activities that once gave them purpose and a sense of importance. For whatever myriad reasons, women appear to cope better with late-life challenges. Perhaps it is because women are often more involved in family-related activities, even if they have had work or professional responsibilities as well.

In the world of retirement planning, one of the recommendations to people to help them avoid feelings of emptiness and loss of purpose is to develop interests and activities while they are still working which they can develop further and enjoy when the work part of their lives is over. I recall visiting one elderly gentleman whose house was full of wonderful woodworked cabinets and furniture. He explained that after he retired, he realized that he would go crazy if he did not have something to do. He had some previous experience with woodworking and decided to enhance his skills with some adult education courses and started redoing his house, resulting in a marvellous dwelling with beautifully crafted items that added not only to the beauty of the house but also to its resale value.

Sam, who had been a practising doctor for almost fifty years, retired ten years ago, against his desires but at the request of his daughter and the advice of his own physician, who felt that it was time for Sam to hang up his shingle. He had very little in the way of outside interests, and when his wife died three years later Sam was quite devastated. For the first few years of retirement, Sam tried to attend medical meetings and see old friends and younger colleagues, but that gradually became very disappointing, as after the few pleasantries about how he was doing and how retirement was treating him, he could not really participate in the world of medical practice, which was often the underlying focus of the meetings. It was clear he liked being called "Doctor," which was understandable, and he enjoyed telling anecdotes, often with great vividness, about his practice and the history of medicine during his time.

I asked him if he liked to write. He answered, "Why did you ask me that? I was actually thinking that maybe I should try doing a bit of a diary, but am not sure who would read it." I told him the story of one of my patients from some years ago who had retired from being the CEO of a large company he owned, and after he stopped working he just fell apart. His wife brought him to me because she was sure he was "losing it," when in fact it was his sense of loss that was giving him the appearance of depression. He had expressed a feeling of worthlessness, and at the age of seventy said he felt it was too soon for it all to be over. Although he liked visiting his children and grandchildren, that family time and the few trips he took with his wife failed to provide much excitement and challenge in his life. He did not like golf very much and, in any event, could not see playing it more than once or twice a month.

As we were talking about his options, he looked over my shoulder at the computer sitting on my desk and said, "I have thought about getting me one of those."

I asked him, "One of what?" as I turned around and realized that he was pointing to my computer. "Why is that?" I followed.

"You know, I was in the British merchant navy during the Second World War. I crossed the Atlantic many times from '41 to '44 and lived through some harrowing times. I was torpedoed, abandoned ship, dealt with U-boats and aircraft attacks and managed to survive even in situations where I lost a lot of my friends from the ship. I have always wanted to tell my story."

"So what is keeping you from doing it? Can you type?" I asked.

He said that although he could not type fast, he could peck on the keyboard because he had worked himself up in his company and at one time did a lot of his own typing when he could not afford a secretary, and his wife, who usually helped him, was busy with their growing family. And then he said, "I am sure I can learn, if I really wanted to."

I responded, "I am sure you can, and I think it is a great idea."

A few months later the retired executive returned with his wife for a follow-up visit. I hardly recognized him when I came into the clinic area, as he appeared engaged and animated as he was registering with the secretary. I looked at his wife, and she smiled at me and nodded in a way that seemed to be positive. When he came into the office, the first thing he said was, "I am up to 1942 and I have been torpedoed for the first time. We haven't been rescued yet. We're still in life boats."

I asked him to elaborate. "I told you I was going to do my memoirs of the merchant navy and the war and my experiences. I've written quite a lot and have reached the first time I was torpedoed. Ships I served on sank twice, and once we were hit but the damage didn't keep us from continuing the trip, sort of limping along. I think I am capturing it all."

He no longer had that sense of having no direction and indicated that he did not care if the book got published, as long as it was there for his family to see whenever they wanted to know more about his life. I wished him well and told him how much I admired him, not only for his war service, but also for putting it all down in print.

After that story, Sam looked at me and said, "You think I should do that as well?"

I nodded yes and told him that I would be happy to look at what he wrote, as it would teach me a bit about the history of medicine in Toronto. I grew up elsewhere and did most of my training elsewhere and much later in time than he did his. He left the office and agreed to think seriously about his new goal and how it might give him something meaningful to do.

Finding meaning in life is very important to every one of us. Family members often recognize when their loved one acts in a way that reflects a loss of that sense: the way they speak, the absence of spark, and the negative commentaries. During our younger and mature adult years, it is the very common and mundane things, mixed with little jewels of insight, delight, and a sense of accomplishment, that make up our lives. When we cook a meal, we want to know that it is good and hope that someone will tell us so. When we get a haircut, we want to hear that our new look is pleasing. These are the kinds of simple but important things that connect people.

There are many ways to bring meaning back into the lives of those we love who, for one reason or another, seem to have lost their spark of interest and excitement. Writing is just one of the many creative ways to excite the mind.

Art, whether painting or sculpture or silkscreening, can do the same, and recognition of this fact has resulted in many artistic activities being offered to seniors, drawing on innate talents and arousing interest in creativity. Outside my office I have two paintings by a woman who in her late seventies began to draw and became an acknowledged late-age artist with pictures hung in many parts of our facility, the two near my office being full of life and spirit and colour.

Music is another way to express one's joy and interest in life and its potential for delight. I have seen music programs for seniors who have significant cognitive impairment and yet can respond very well to sounds, rhythms, and melodies that evoke wonderful feelings from their past. There are choirs in which seniors excel, and the need to be at a place for rehearsal and performance can be a very strong motivating force that gives excitement and a sense of satisfaction to an older person.

My own mother continued to participate in dance until just before her final illness. Involved in dance since her adolescent years, she always found a way to dance at any gathering where it was possible. She joined groups of folk dancers and, if given a chance, was happy to perform to bring joy to others. During her final days, after her devastating stroke, one of the first ways she showed any movement of her paralyzed leg was to move her toes to music that I provided to her through earphones and to point her toe in the way she would when she demonstrated a ballet step.

There are many ways to be creative besides participating in the arts, music, and writing. For some, gardening might do it, and for others photography or flower arranging. It does not matter what one chooses to do, as long as it draws on one's sense of creativity. It should also be something that one can share with family and friends and evoke the kind of feedback and encouragement that gives meaning and satisfaction.

One man I knew loved to make small wooden toys and items for his grandchildren. Nothing gave him more joy than seeing them play with something he made or hearing one his granddaughters tell a friend that the little chairs they were sitting on were made by her grandpa. My mother started making kitchen aprons in her seventies and would bring one to every household she visited when she wanted to give a personal gift. Years after her death, I still see them on relatives to whom she gave one long ago, and nothing is lovelier that to hear them extol the beauty, usefulness, and love that came with those aprons because they were made by someone for whom they cared.

Children can help their parents find their creative spirit in many ways. When possible, they should provide opportunities for their parents to participate in creative activities and share their joy of accomplishment — that is all any of us want from our lives: to do things that have meaning and thereby give meaning to our lives.

SIBLINGS:

In Charge and On the Attack

When brothers and sisters vie for attention and favour from an elderly parent, the inevitable outcome is sibling rivalry and mutual distrust. If ever there is a time for siblings to pull together, it's when a parent is in failing health.

THE CHALLENGE

Edna Delaney lives in a retirement home in Vancouver. She's a vigorous, high-energy eighty-six-year-old, but she is showing early signs of dementia that he doctor says is likely Alzheimer's disease. She's been highly independent since the death of her husband, Frank. From the time he suffered a massive heart attack, Edna blossomed in terms of managing his care and their family finances. Three years after his heart attack, and after steadily declining health, Frank died. Edna grieved greatly, and then she seemed to put Frank's death, but not her ongoing love of him, behind her, and decided she wanted to live what was left of her life to the fullest.

Edna has four children: Frank Jr., fifty-seven, a lawyer who specializes in estate planning and lives with his family in nearby Burnaby; Joan, fifty-three, a housewife who lives with her family in Victoria; Roger, fifty-one, divorced and living in Los Angeles where he works as an on-again, off-again scriptwriter for various television shows; and Heather, fifty, who lives with her second husband and their three children in Ottawa, where she sells real estate.

When their father died, there was some discussion among the four siblings of the best way to help their mother. It was agreed that Frank Jr. and Joan would take lead roles, since they were in closest proximity to their mother. Both Roger and Heather pledged to help as needed.

About six months after his father was buried, Frank Jr. talked with his mother about what help she felt she really needed and what other help she wanted. In that discussion, Edna made it clear that she wanted to remain as independent as possible and not rely on her children. However, she also made it clear that she wanted to stay in touch with them on a regular basis. She said she favoured none over the other, and that she felt that they were all equal in terms of her affection and attention.

Financially, Edna is in extremely good condition. Her husband was very successful in real estate and in the stock market, and Edna's net worth is somewhere in the area of $3.5 million. The greater concern — at least on the surface — is her health and well-being.

All four Delaney children have a pretty good idea of their mother's financial worth. Frank Jr. has a high income that he's invested wisely, and he is the least concerned about any possible inheritance. Roger, in contrast, is the most financially insecure, because his work is sporadic while his lifestyle is pretty expensive, and he's very aware of what a good inheritance could do for his life.

During the past year, Edna has become increasingly confused, uncertain, and forgetful. She's fallen several times in her apartment, lying on the floor until either the maid service found her or it was noticed that she wasn't present in the dining room for a meal. Although she has been given a panic button to wear around her neck to use in precisely such situations, Edna — either in her stubborn wish for independence or because of her forgetfulness — more often than not leaves the button in her night table drawer.

Because of these experiences, the administrator at Edna's retirement home called Frank Jr. a few weeks ago and explained that his mother required more attention than the home could offer. He suggested that Frank consider how to ensure she gets the level of attention that she increasingly seems to need. They discussed increasing the care provided on-site with some in-home supplementary services and even a move to a nursing home, which they both believe she would strongly resist.

In addition, a few weeks ago during Edna's annual physical examination, her doctor surmised, based on her movements and a slight tilt to one side, that she may have had a mild stroke. The doctor has scheduled her for a CT scan to see if there is any evidence to support the observations.

But the doctor did tell Edna — and also called Frank Jr. to advise him — that there could be other smaller strokes and that there is a potential for a more serious stroke to occur because of Edna's weight, eating habits, and past history of heavy smoking.

Frank Jr. shared this information with his brother and sisters. They all agreed at the time that he should take the lead in ensuring their mother has the care that she needs. Based on this collective decision, Frank Jr. has decided that his mother needs more in-home help. He has arranged for her to be moved to a larger apartment in the retirement home and has hired a caregiver, with backup support. In all, Edna's accommodation, meals, and care are now costing nearly $7,000 a month.

Edna has been prescribed medications to improve her function and decrease the likelihood of further strokes, and Frank Jr. has arranged for the pills to be dispensed in such a way that Edna will be more likely to take them correctly. The increase in help is imperative now that her medication regimen is more complex and her care needs are increasing.

Roger, who seldom called or visited his mother in the past, now calls her every other day. He has visited her twice in the past six months.

Edna confides to Frank Jr. that Roger has suggested that she should move to California to be near him. Roger has also impressed on his mother that the weather there would be better for her. Plus, in all his calls, Roger has probed about her will — again, something Edna tells Frank Jr. — and has urged her to consider which of her children needs and deserves more of her money when she passes away.

Frank Jr., having reflected on all he's been told and has learned, urges his mother to think through what she wants to do with her will, which hasn't been revised since before her husband died. But he's reluctant to give advice. Despite his vocation, it's an uncomfortable situation for Frank Jr. since this isn't just a client — it's his mother. Heather, in her weekly telephone call, urges her mother to write a new will and plan her life to suit her own level of comfort and needs, pointing out that all her children are adults and can and should look after themselves without any longer depending on her. Finally, Joan, who visits her mother once a month, is subtly lobbying her mother by reminding Edna that she's always there for her and that she comes to see her regularly.

When Frank Jr. conducts a mental inventory of the state of the family affairs, he realizes that none of Edna's children are really talking to the others about the situation and how best to manage it. He's troubled by this, but not quite certain what to do about it. While Frank is busy with his day-to-day work and thinking about how to talk with his mother, Roger arrives for another visit. During that weekend, Roger applies great pressure on Edna to move to Los Angeles and to give him power of attorney over her financial affairs and her health needs. He vows to look after her, telling his mother that he's the only one who doesn't have family to support and, therefore, he can devote his time and attention to her well-being.

Edna tells Frank Jr. about Roger's thoughtful suggestion. But she's already confused, and when Frank Jr. tells her to think about what's best for her, she confides that Roger made it clear that he was the one who could care for her best, and that the American health care system would do more for her.

A week later, Roger calls his brother and sisters and makes his case for being the prime caregiver and moving their mother to Los Angeles. He's adamant in his position and pleads for support. Heather is concerned, worried that Roger has a self-serving agenda. Joan doesn't know what to think, except that Roger is going to end up with a lot of money. And Frank Jr. is worried that his mother will give in to the pressure being exerted by Roger.

None of the siblings feels comfortable with the others or with the way things are shaping up. Nor do any of them know what to do, or how to do it, except for Roger, who the others believe has a clear agenda.

Suddenly, there is growing doubt and concern among them and a sense that perhaps they must jockey for their mother's attention and favour.

THE HEALTH CARE PROFESSIONAL'S POINT OF VIEW

The primary focus of all of these deliberations must be Edna. If any of the children forget this, there must be a way of reminding them clearly, while things are still reasonably stable and before there is a crisis in Edna's care needs or a breakdown in the relationship of the siblings. This may require a family meeting, even if it means that all of them have to visit Vancouver. If that is impossible, they should plan a conference call in which they all can participate. If their basic relationship prior to Edna's decline has been good, they can build upon that foundation to take the steps that will assure Edna's well-being for the present and the future.

There are a number of issues that must be aired during the family discussion. With the necessary information from the doctor (a family meeting with the doctor could be of great value, but might not be logistically possible), it should be possible to get a prognosis and likely timeline of the progression of Edna's medical condition.

If she has Alzheimer's disease and also suffers from some small strokes, it is pretty clear that there will be continued deterioration of her mental and intellectual functioning. This is the case even if she is considered a suitable candidate for one of the new drugs now used in combatting Alzheimer's disease (e.g., Aricipt®, Exelon®, or Reminyl®) which might decrease the rate of decline but will not offer anything like a cure for her condition.

With the knowledge that there will be a progressive decline, the next question that must be asked is whether, in fact, Edna has the mental capacity to make the kinds of decisions that she is being asked to make, such as changing her will or moving to California. It is likely that if formally tested, she would be found not to have the capacity to change her will in any substantive way. If she were to make changes now, they would likely be open to legal challenge after she dies if one of the siblings is not happy with the changes.

If she is not mentally capable of making a new will, it is also unlikely that she can understand and appreciate the implications of a move to California or of making what would be considered a legally capable decision. Also it should be made clear to all the siblings, especially Roger, that as their mother deteriorates her care needs will increase and she will need a lot of family support, which is unlikely to be available from Roger alone in Los Angeles.

As for the quality of care that Edna may eventually require, she should be able to get as good if not better long-term care at a much lower cost in Vancouver than in Los Angeles. The cost factor should be considered if there is concern about her having the funds to sustain her over a long period of decline and perhaps leave a legacy for her children, which seems to be her wish.

With these factors taken into consideration, the siblings' discussion should include who is going to be the formal spokesperson for the family so that decisions about her health can be made. Unless they agree to a spokesperson to represent them (with, of course, reasonable consultation with the others), they could end up in a situation in which the courts appoint a guardian in the absence of a defined decision-maker.

If the family decides, as most families do, that it is better for them to find a way to co-operate than to have an outside person make decisions without their consultation, they will eventually agree to designate one of them, likely Frank Jr., to be the decision-maker (surrogate). It would have been better if, prior to Edna's losing her capacity, she and her children had discussed the possibilities for the future should she become ill. At that time they could have agreed on this process and structure, rather than leaving it open to potential conflict that may result in resentment among the children as Edna deteriorates.

Assuming that, after hearing the facts and implications of the various options, the children agree that the best arrangement for Edna is to have her stay in Vancouver with Frank Jr. taking the primary care role, they then need to make some backup arrangements. They should agree that when Frank Jr. needs time to go on a vacation or travel on business, someone else will be in Vancouver to ensure that Edna continues her social visits and outings.

With this agreement in place, it is possible that Frank Jr. will be able to carry on with the main responsibility. Rather than challenging his role, his siblings should be grateful that they have him as a strong support for Edna and not someone who is likely motivated by a future inheritance.

If the situation is not resolved happily, and Roger or one of the other siblings challenges the status quo, it might be necessary for Frank Jr. to go to court and ask that he be appointed the formal surrogate and power of attorney for Edna's financial and personal needs. It is likely that he would be successful in such a request, but the repercussions in terms of family structure and resentment could be so great that the fabric of the family would be irrevocably destroyed. If the children feel inclined to pursue the matter through legal channels, they would be wise to get some impartial advice on the short- and long-term implications for them, for Edna, and for their family relationships.

If the family agrees to Frank Jr.'s role as primary caregiver, they can all focus on making sure that Edna receives the best possible health care as she continues to decline mentally and physically. This will be provided through the co-operation of a loving and devoted family who do their best to make her comfortable and to visit as often as possible, considering that some of the children live far away. Whatever financial legacy might be left to them, the most important legacy is the knowledge that they cared for their mother, taking into account her best interests and not their own.

THE CONFLICTED SINGLE CHILD:

A Confusing Battle of Priorities

What does a young, single, upwardly mobile woman do when her mother is in the early stages of dementia and rejects all attempts to offer support? The emerging frustration has the potential to harm both the relationship and her career.

THE CHALLENGE

Maria Pontes is thirty-three years old. She is single and lives in an upscale downtown apartment building. Maria has been with a large, multinational public relations/public affairs firm for four years and is considered a shining star with high potential.

A political science graduate from Carleton University, she completed an MBA at York University five years ago. She is ambitious, assertive, articulate, and knows a bright future is in her grasp. Maria works extremely hard, putting in long hours on weekdays and at least five to ten hours most weekends. She also has a fairly active social life and is an avid squash player, trying to get in three or four hits a week, usually early in the morning.

Maria's most significant current challenge is her mother, Camilla. Camilla is sixty-seven years of age. She moved to Canada from Portugal when she was thirty-one with her husband, Manuel. They settled in Hamilton, where Manuel worked at one of the steel mills and Camilla worked at a small fabricating shop. She had difficulty conceiving and had almost given up when she finally became pregnant. Maria was born, and no other pregnancies followed, which was a bit of a disappointment for both Manuel and Camilla.

When Maria was fifteen, the family took a trip to Portugal, where she got to meet for the first time her grandparents and relatives. The trip left a lasting impression on Maria; she learned all about her family and discovered they were very warm and caring. She was a hit with her aunts and uncles and found the basis for what would be a strong long-distance relationship with them and her six cousins.

In fact, from that visit on, she has corresponded with her cousins, first by mail and during the past few years by email, in English, since their broken English was and remains much better than her fractured Portuguese.

When Maria was seventeen years old, her father died of a brain aneurysm. She and her mother grieved for Manuel deeply and for a long time. Both loved him very much. Maria had actually been closer to her father than to her mother. No matter how tired he was after a long shift at the plant, he would spend time with Maria, teaching her all he knew and always encouraging her to strive for an education as the means to success. He often reminded Maria that they were immigrants to Canada from poor but very decent, honest, and hard-working families. He told her that she would be the first generation to break through the barriers they all had lived with for generations and challenged her to study hard, to have high goals, and never to doubt herself. Maria valued her father's convictions and truly cherished his vision of what she could do with her life.

Maria and her father also shared a passion for hockey. Throughout her childhood and until his death, watching Saturday night hockey on television had been a ritual for them. Two or three times a season, they would go to Toronto to see the Maple Leafs play.

So when Manual suddenly died, it was crushing for Maria. She faltered at school and became withdrawn. Her mother, while also in pain, sometimes became agitated with Maria's behaviour and admonished her for being so hard on herself.

Eventually, Maria came to terms with her father's death and plunged full steam into her schoolwork. She graduated with honours and won two scholarships, and the rest, as she likes to say, is just life playing out as it should.

When she landed her current job, she commuted for the first year and lived with her mother. Then she moved to Toronto, explaining to her mother that the demands of her job meant that the daily travel time was simply too much. Camilla was upset, and after six months, Maria encouraged her to move closer. Her mother did part-time work as a salesperson at a department store and could find a similar job in Toronto.

Camilla resisted for another six months and then decided to move to Scarborough, at the eastern end of the city. She found a small but suitable apartment with Maria's help, moved, and within two months got a full-time job at a new big box outlet.

Maria tried hard to see her mother two or three times a week, at least one of those times being for a home-cooked meal. The relationship, though, was strained. Her mother wasn't very happy with the move because most of her friends were in Hamilton. More than that, while Camilla never articulated it she was, in fact, unhappy that Maria didn't spend the same kind of time with her now that she remembered Maria spending with her father. And she had a hard time understanding exactly what Maria did, or why she worked such long hours.

Two years ago, Camilla seemed to start changing in ways Maria didn't understand. The changes were very subtle at first: her mother would call to ask for something and then, when Maria did what she had asked, her mother would act surprised and deny asking in the first place. Sometimes when Maria arrived for dinner and a visit, her mother wouldn't have any dinner prepared. But Maria was busy with her work and personal life and never thought much about it.

However, six to eight months ago, Maria noticed more worrisome changes that started to concern her. Her mother seemed to be both more withdrawn and more combative. Camilla started asking for more help, yet whenever Maria tried to be helpful, her mother would berate her or deny asking. She stopped calling Maria at the office, and while they used to speak for at least a few minutes most evenings, now it was only once or twice a week. When she visited, Maria noticed that her mother's apartment wasn't as neat and tidy as it used to be, and her mother seemed somewhat more confused as she spoke. Plus, Camilla was now working part-time, only about a dozen hours a week. Maria also noted that some bills were not paid on time, and one month the phone company called a few times to question what was going on with the late bill payment.

Maria got worried. She finally insisted that her mother have a full medical examination, and even went with her. The physician's conclusion: Camilla was physically well, but she was exhibiting symptoms of early Alzheimer's disease. Camilla denied that there was anything wrong with her.

The doctor explained that there were a number of drugs that could help Camilla. He prescribed a new medication for her, and while she got the medication, Maria discovered she wasn't taking it. On a visit to her mother, she looked in the medicine cabinet and saw the container was still full.

The doctor also recommended that her mother attend a day program a few times a week that helped people with Alzheimer's understand how to cope with their disease and served as a mutual help network. Camilla flatly refused to attend.

Meanwhile, Maria was finding she had less and less time for her mother, or anything else except work. While she used to be able to squeeze in time to take her mother for doctors' appointments and shopping, it was becoming more difficult to get away at a reasonable time.

Now, Maria is conflicted. The president of her company's Canadian operations met with her and said a promotion was in the works. Her new position would require extensive travel across Canada to manage a major account and would probably mean that she'd be reassigned to Amsterdam within the next year to work on the global team managing the strategy and hands-on support at the client's head office.

Maria wants to help and support her mother, but she is also eager to take on the new position: it fulfills the dream her father had instilled in her. She's considered all the possible options and decided that perhaps getting her mother back to Portugal would be the best solution, especially if she would be working in Europe anyway; after all, she could find time to visit her there more easily than in Toronto. And her mother would be with her family, with all the support that offered. She even phoned her cousins to talk about this option, and the word back was that the family would be more than pleased to have Camilla return home and to help her.

But Camilla flatly rejected the idea of a move back to her home-town. She lashed out at Maria, accusing her of wanting to get her out of the way. She also accused Maria of wanting to take her money and started withdrawing substantial sums of money from the bank; Maria knew because the account is a joint one and she can access it online. She has spoken to the bank manager about her concerns.

Meanwhile, when Maria visits Camilla, she notices yet more evidence that her mother seems to be neglecting her home and herself. And she experiences more strain in their relationship— more tension, more terse words and accusations. Maria wants to do the right thing, for her mother and for herself, but all she sees is conflict, confusion, and uncertainty.

THE HEALTH CARE PROFESSIONAL'S POINT OF VIEW

Doing the right thing for one's parent is not always what neatly fits into one's personal or professional aspirations. There is always a balance, and depending on many factors, a child may move in one direction rather than another. Despite the difficulties with the relationship between Maria and Camilla when she was growing up, and especially after her father died, Maria does not sound like she is willing to abandon her mother for her career or personal life.

The challenge, then, is how to provide for her mother in a way that can assure some semblance of safety and security while she tries to pursue both a personal and a professional life. The fact that her mother refuses to acknowledge her illness is very common in diseases such as Alzheimer's. But until such time that she is clearly a threat to herself or others, it would be very difficult to take over or force care on her mother. Some simple steps can be taken to make sure that bills are paid — Maria can arrange automatic withdrawals for utility and other necessary payments — even though Camilla may resent Maria's appearing to take over.

As for Camilla's withdrawing money from her bank account, that may be a bit more complicated and touchy. Since it is a joint account, Maria can likely put a limit on how much money can be withdrawn at any given time, although Camilla might get upset with the bank teller who refuses to give her whatever amount she demands. Maria will then have to explain the reason for the limit and deal with Camilla's anger. If the account were not a joint one, it could be necessary for Maria to take the step of using the legal system to verify that Camilla suffers from dementia and requires Maria to be a surrogate for some decisions, including financial ones. This may be necessary eventually, but since in this case the account is already joint in nature that legal step can probably be avoided for now.

Maria cannot force Camilla into a day program, and in some ways, unless her condition becomes severe and it is deemed that she does not have the mental capacity to make any decisions, there is not much that Maria can do. Medications cannot be forced upon her, and future visits to the doctor may be refused as well. If Camilla thinks that the doctor and Maria are in cahoots, she may refuse further visits and therefore decline any offers of treatment. Certainly she will not attend a day program for support if she denies there is a problem. Many people in such circumstances will leave a program for Alzheimer's disease patients when they sense that everyone is worse than they are and deny that they have any need for such a program.

In a case like this, when the parent refuses help and the dementia has not yet progressed to the point that a surrogate for decision-making can be appointed, sometimes the only thing a family can do is wait for some terrible crises to occur. The challenge for Maria, even if she does become Camilla's surrogate, is whether she is willing to force her mother to do something that she does not want to do. Their lifelong pattern of interaction was always based on her mother having very strong opinions and a very strong will and Maria usually backing down in times of conflict. She does not think she would be prepared to take the opposite position unless things were really terrible, which is not the case.

In fact, other than the bill payment issue, which can be dealt with, and the withdrawal of money, Camilla does manage. Work is an issue, and it looks like she will be let go as soon as she makes too many errors and misses days of work too often. Maria has spoken to the supervisor, who was very understanding and agreed to let Camilla go with a good excuse and a send-off party to make her feel good. Camilla seems to shop for her personal items adequately, though Maria sometimes finds excess amounts of some products in the refrigerator, suggesting that Camilla may be forgetting what she has bought, but this is not a big problem so far. Maria does get calls from her mother from time to time about matters that have already been discussed or decided upon, but she has learned from her meetings with the Alzheimer's Society how to deal with those repeated calls. Maria also notes that Camilla reverts more often to Portuguese, and Maria must struggle to respond, as her command of the language, which was not her mother tongue but rather the one she heard spoken around the house, is marginal.

The real problems for Maria are long-term planning for Camilla and what to do with her own career. Getting her mother back to Portugal on face value sounds like a good idea, and with a large, accepting, and loving family that is willing to take this on, one might have jumped at the opportunity. However, if Camilla does not want to go, at least at this stage of her life, it would be very hard to force her to travel home. Maria might try to convince her to take a trip back to visit, with the hope that once there she will feel all the emotional ties to her native country and her family and agree to stay. But if that is not possible, sending her to Portugal for the time being does not seem to be a viable option. Maria must consider just how close Camilla is to these relatives in Portugal now that she has lived for some many years in Canada. If she has few contacts and a limited network in Toronto, and has kept some closeness with her family back home, this might turn out to be the ultimate answer to the problem, but it will have to unfold with time, as it cannot readily be forced.

Another option is to ask one or more of the Portuguese family to visit Toronto and stay with or close to Camilla so that she can relate to them and hopefully develop an attachment that might encourage her to consider the possibility of returning home, first for a visit and then maybe with the plan to remain there. If this were part of a plan, Maria would have to work closely with the relatives in Portugal to try to develop the supportive and caring environment that might lead Maria to think that a trip back would be a good thing, rather than something being forced on her by her ungrateful daughter.

As for Maria's career, she might have to discuss with her boss the realities of her life. It may not be possible for her to take on the overseas job until things have been settled with her mother. There are many sacrifices that children can make in order to care for their parents. Children must accept that no one can plan for what will be; the real challenge in a caring relationship is how one deals with situations one cannot control. It is hard to imagine that Maria would leave Camilla to fend for herself while she takes on an overseas portfolio. In all likelihood the plan would fail and she would have to return home as things deteriorated. Rather than undertaking such a move now, she might have to defer it, even at the risk of her career path for the time being, in order to be a dutiful and caring daughter. In an era in which many highly qualified workers face similar problems with aging parents, it is likely that if Maria explains the situation to her boss, some alternative career path can be worked out. She is clearly good at what she does, and most people in organizations value excellent people and invest in them long-term. So this may be a time for the company to support Maria so that she can be everything she might be for them in the future.

Being a single child of a parent with dementia is not easy. Not having other siblings to share the responsibilities and decision-making challenges is difficult. But there are ways to get help. On the advice of Camilla's doctor, Maria joined the Alzheimer's Society and finds the meetings and newsletters and other publications very useful. Speaking to other families who are struggling with similar issues really is a support for Maria. The doctor also arranged a few meetings with a social worker to assist Maria in figuring out what her options are, and she has found comfort in having someone to whom she can vent and express her innermost concerns. The doctor suggested that if Maria needs more intensive support, she should consider getting herself to a psychologist or other counsellor to help her work through her relationship with Camilla and to explore how her needs and those of her mother interconnect.

In situations such as this one, something usually happens that helps to resolve the issue. Sometimes, unfortunately, it is a crisis, such as an illness that makes things worse, that forces a certain direction of decision-making. Maybe Camilla agrees to visit her family and decides that it would be best to stay, or a family member visits from Portugal and Camilla agrees to return for a visit and then remains there. Many things can happen. The important point is that Maria has to be supported in her quest to do the right thing personally and hopefully get the support she needs at her workplace so she realizes that ultimately she will be able to fulfill her career goals and dreams while at the same time being the caring and dutiful daughter that she is.

THE STROKE:
Sudden Challenges and Changes

A self-sufficient parent suffers a series of strokes, creating an instant family crisis requiring careful co-ordination of care and attention.

THE CHALLENGE

Diane is fifty-one years old and married to Terry, who is fifty-five. They have an eighteen-year-old daughter, Amanda. This is Terry's second marriage. He divorced his first wife after fifteen years of an unhappy and acrimonious marriage that produced a daughter, Jill, who is twenty-three years old and lives on her own.

Diane's father left her mother, Wilma, more than a decade ago. A quick divorce followed, and he hasn't been heard from since. Diane, while never close to her father or approving of his lifestyle and treatment of her mother, still on occasion wonders about him.

Terry lost both of his parents in a fatal automobile accident six years ago while they were on their way to a vacation in Florida.

Because both Diane and Terry were the only children in their families, neither of them has any close family to speak of, other than a few distant cousins and an uncle out west. That's why they are so close to Diane's mother.

Until recently, Wilma lived on her own in a large, rambling house, an hour's drive in the country from Diane and Terry's home in Saskatoon. She'd lived there ever since her husband had left her. Wilma had never remarried, but for the past five or six years she has been casually seeing a widower who lived not far from her; they were just good friends (or so it seemed) who enjoyed being together.

Diane often drove out to visit her mother just for an hour or so. Diane and Terry also regularly visited Wilma, with a protesting Amanda in tow. Not that Amanda didn't like her grandmother; she was just at an age when she would rather spend all her time with her friends and not her parents. However, despite not wanting to go — especially for weekend visits — Amanda usually had a reasonably good time once she got there. And Wilma, who at seventy-two years of age was full of energy, would take the bus to the city and visit for several days at a time with her daughter and family.

Wilma had always been in good health. The first time in her life that she'd been in the hospital was four years ago for a day surgery cataract procedure. She faithfully went to her annual medical checkups, and she always fared well in the final assessments. Her one big problem was her weight. Wilma loved her food and loved to eat. She was about fifty pounds overweight, and no amount of frequent but loosely applied dieting got her weight down.

On one of her short visits to see her mother, Diane observed that Wilma was talking with a slight slur and that she leaned to one side in a way that she hadn't noticed before. But for all intents and purposes, Wilma seemed to be fine, just as full of energy as ever. Diane asked her mother if she was feeling all right, and Wilma assured her she couldn't be better. Yet something kept nagging at Diane, and she pressured her mother to make an appointment to see her doctor.

Two days later, Diane called her mother in the morning — a time she was always home — and there was no answer. Troubled, she called Wilma's friend, who said he hadn't seen her in a couple of days. After getting no answer a few more times, Diane called one of Wilma's neighbours and asked if she'd look to see if her mother was there. She wasn't.

Worried, Diane cancelled her next two meetings and drove to her mother's house. Just as she arrived, there was Wilma getting out of the local taxi. Wilma explained that she'd been to see her doctor, who wondered if she might have suffered a very small stoke. But, her mother said, everything seemed to be all right, although the doctor did suggest that she needed a good going over. And that's how Diane happened to be there when, an hour later, her mother toppled out of her chair, unable to speak or move. Diane managed to help Wilma to the car and drove to the small local hospital.

Her doctor was summoned. He confirmed she'd had another stroke and that this one was substantial. He arranged to transfer Wilma to the larger regional hospital.

The next two days were a terrible blur for Diane. She was told that her mother had suffered a massive stroke. Wilma's entire right side was immobile, and she initially lost all ability to speak. After the first day, she could communicate, but with only a few halting words. Terry was shaken and Amanda was in tears. Even Jill, who didn't feel a great deal of closeness to Diane's mother, was moved to ask how she might help.

Diane arranged for her mother to be transported to a hospital in the city, where she could get more sophisticated care and diagnostic tests, and where she'd be closer to the family. A week later, Wilma was transferred again — this time to a rehabilitation hospital as a temporary measure. By now, although Wilma could utter a handful of words, it was clear from all the medical advice Diane had managed to collect that her mother probably would never walk again and certainly couldn't live on her own.

Wilma was on a regimen of daily therapy sessions, which seemed to help somewhat, but there was no significant improvement. Nor was there any further deterioration in her condition. All in all, Wilma was holding her own, and she was trying to be as co-operative as possible.

Since entering the rehabilitation hospital, Wilma has had yet another stroke, albeit a much smaller one. She is now totally dependent on full-time care and assistance. She can't walk at all, and she has lost all use of her right arm. She is unable to move out of her bed or wheelchair without help. She has also developed some problems with swallowing and eating and occasionally chokes on her food. A nutritionist has made some recommendations about positioning her when she eats and setting the pace of feeding as well as modifying the consistency of foods.

Totally unprepared for this devastating event, Diane and Terry wonder what they should do next to help Wilma and make her as comfortable as possible. They aren't certain where Wilma could live. They recognize that, even though they have a small guest room in their house, Diane's mother needs a level of attention that they can't provide, and they have no room for a full-time caregiver. They also know they have limited time because of their job pressures, and limited resources because they paid for Amanda to go to a private school and now she attends university in the United States. However, they do want to do the right thing for Wilma.

THE HEALTH CARE PROFESSIONAL'S POINT OF VIEW

Diane and her family must ask themselves, "What is the right thing to do?" The main focus should be deciding where Wilma will get the best care for her immediate and long-term needs and what the family can reasonably do under their present living circumstances. While it might be the ideal situation for Wilma to move in with her family, it would be a monumental undertaking and also a very expensive one. They would have to renovate the house to accommodate Wilma's needs and arrange for full-time help. The cost of twenty-four-hour-a-day care is prohibitive for most families, unless they are very well off financially. This is not the situation with Diane and Terry, who are, in fact, struggling with their own financial situation now that their daughter is in university.

If keeping Wilma at home is not a viable option, the only other choice is to find a suitable long-term care facility. They can look for a facility either near where they live or near Wilma's own home. They need to weigh the importance of Wilma being near her social network of friends and neighbours against the convenience of being nearer to the family, who will be Wilma's main support.

Assuming that Wilma is not able to communicate, it may be necessary for her family to try to explore who among her friends might really be available to visit her. If the only important person is her male friend from her neighbourhood, they might speak to him about how they can arrange for him to visit her from time to time. Perhaps they could either periodically pick him up or arrange for his transportation so that he could spend an afternoon at Wilma's nursing home and make a nice visit out of it. Wilma may or may not be able to recognize or fully interact with her friend, but if they could continue some kind of a meaningful relationship, it is worth pursuing this avenue for her benefit.

The rest of the visiting will be up to the family. Although it is not easy, they should try to develop plans that will make each visit a bit special. For example, they might bring some treats that are appropriate for Wilma. Of course, if they bring food, it is important to make sure that it is something that she can eat, especially since she has some swallowing difficulties. If Wilma likes flowers, it may be worth putting some plants in her room, as long as someone will take care of them. Taking pictures to share with Wilma would be a very nice way to keep her up to date with family events. Going for a walk around the premises is often a special event for nursing home residents and is generally something staff cannot do frequently. Some families hire private companions to take their loved one on an outing or walk once in awhile depending on the situation. If the staff thinks it is safe, going for a drive or some other kind of outing might also be a nice way to bring something new and special into Wilma's life. If music is something special for her, they should arrange for a CD player or tape machine for her room that she can listen to whenever she wants.

This would also be a very good time for Diane and Terry to explore with Wilma what she would like to happen should things take a turn for the worse. For example, if Wilma has strong views about end-of-life issues based on deep-seated personal or religious reasons, these should be confirmed. If it is thought that she would prefer not to have heroic treatments provided, this should be established as reasonably as possible.

The issue of feeding tubes might also be considered in view of the problems that Wilma is already experiencing with her eating. These issues should be presented in a way that does not frighten Wilma, as an assurance that nothing will be done for her or to her that she would not want if she could express her wishes herself.

If effective communication takes place, it may be possible for Diane and Terry to understand reasonably the limits and boundaries of care that Wilma would prefer if she were able to communicate at the time. So, for example, if she gets an infection, she would want to be treated if there were a good chance of full recovery. But she might prefer to not have cardiopulmonary resuscitation in the event of a cardiac arrest, or she may not want a permanent feeding tube should she not be able to eat normally. Knowing Wilma's wishes now, when her condition is stable and non-threatening, would certainly make it much easier for Diane and Terry to live with what are often difficult decisions at a time of crisis.

These are not easy times. But with the goodwill and dedication that appear to be motivating Diane and her husband, and with a bit of luck, Wilma should be able to manage reasonably well for some time in the nursing home, perhaps months to years. She might even improve in terms of function for a while, but then inevitably something will occur from which she cannot recover. Diane and Terry should be ready for all eventualities and be thankful for any period of comfort and enjoyment that Wilma can experience during this very difficult period of her life.

DEMENTIA AND DEPRESSION:

Reading the Signs

*Discovering that a parent has
significant health problems but is in
total denial is a disturbing and often
frightening experience for children.
Such a stressful situation requires
careful action to best help all involved.*

THE CHALLENGE

Al and Denise Wilson have been married for forty-five years. Al is seventy-two years old, and Denise is sixty-eight. They've both been in excellent health all their lives.

Al retired at age sixty-five on a full pension after working with the same company since completing university. At about the same time, Denise opted to take a downsizing severance package at the company where she'd been a secretary for more than thirty years, and this provided her with a good pension also.

Al, a structural engineer with a mid-sized consulting company, was actually relieved to retire when he did. He'd found the last couple of years at the office to be increasingly difficult. What bothered Al was that periodically, sometimes for a number of months at a time, he found he was having a hard time concentrating on his assignments, and the more complex a job was, the longer it took him to complete it. He never mentioned this to anyone, and he told himself it was because he was bored and tired after so many years of doing the same thing. He also had periods when he had problems sleeping, and so he attributed his lack of concentration to his periodic lack of sleep. Al also thought part of the problem may be that he was eagerly anticipating retirement.

After considering what they really wanted to do in their golden years, Al and Denise sold their comfortable home in Toronto and moved into a retirement community on the shores of a lake north of the city.

The transition, which worried them a bit, went very smoothly. As they're still fond of telling people they meet, they both adjusted "like a duck to water"; they had no second thoughts and certainly no regrets. They've thoroughly enjoyed their lifestyle in their new home. They cultivated friendships with a number of other retired couples, played bridge weekly, and, best of all, golfed every other day. Last year, they splurged and bought a small sailboat and took some lessons. During the summer months they sailed most evenings for an hour on the lake.

For the past several years, Al and Denise have spent six weeks each winter in Florida at a condominium they share with another couple they've known for years. All in all, Al and Denise are very much enjoying their lives and feel that the years of work and careful savings are paying off handsomely.

Their only child, Mary, is thirty-seven years old and lives in Toronto with her husband, Bob, and their two children, Amy, who is seventeen, and Tom, who is fourteen. Mary and her family are close to her parents and visit them about once every two weeks — sometimes staying for a weekend. Most holidays are spent together.

Bob's parents live in North Bay and both are in good health. Twice a year his parents come to visit them in Toronto, and at least annually they trek to North Bay to visit for a few days. And, of course, they all talk to one another on the telephone regularly.

For all intents and purposes, all the family members honestly like one another and get along well.

About four months ago, Denise noticed for the first time that Al was "not his old self," as she described it to Mary at the time. He seemed to be more withdrawn, she told Mary, and sometimes indecisive about things like what to eat — something about which he'd always had very fixed views, with strong likes and dislikes.

Mary forgot about what her mother told her, and Denise herself put it somewhere on the back burner of her mind for the time.

As the weeks passed, Denise realized that her husband was spending less and less time in his small woodworking shop that he'd equipped in part of the garage. Finally, she asked him about it. Al said he'd just lost interest in woodworking, that it was too time-consuming and too hard.

Yet Denise knew Al truly enjoyed making small pieces of furniture and prided himself on the detailed work. That's why a few days later she asked about his woodworking again, this time to enquire when he'd finally build her the shelves above the washer and dryer. Al became very agitated. He said he didn't know when he might have the time to build the shelves. When Denise reminded him that he had all the time in the world, Al didn't respond. So the subject was dropped.

Then, just a few weeks later, Al changed his mind about going for their usual after-dinner sail, and he did so again a week later. This was definitely not like Al at all, because he loved that little boat and the feel of the breeze on the lake. Denise asked him if something was wrong, and Al said, no, he just didn't feel like sailing these days, as he had some increased pain in his back, the result of an old athletic injury. He claimed that sailing seemed a bit risky for him and that he worries more about their safety out on the water. He seemed even more irritated when she asked again about the shelves. He told her that if she needed the shelves so badly, she should just go out and buy some.

Not long after that conversation, Mary, Bob, Amy, and Tom came for a one-day visit. It was a sunny, warm day and everyone wanted to go sailing, but Al said he didn't feel like it — and that was a first. Mary asked her father several times but got the same negative response every time.

During the course of the day, Denise pulled her daughter aside and told her about her father's recent change of behaviour and how it was confusing to her. Mary was mystified. She watched her father very closely for the rest of the visit. She noticed that he sometimes appeared withdrawn, as if he were in his own world. He did not laugh in his usual way at her husband's wisecracks and puns, which was out of character. She mentioned this to her mother later on that evening, who said that this kind of behaviour had been occurring quite often lately. Mary asked if there was anything else, and her mother admitted that Al was no longer interested in sex; whenever she approached him he found an excuse for not participating, usually complaining of fatigue or backache, a problem that he had had for years but that had never before interfered with what had been, up until a few months ago, a very satisfying sex life for the two of them.

Later Mary told her husband about her observations and her mother's comments, and he suggested that they should both see a doctor for a good assessment.

The next day, Mary called her mother and asked when her parents had last had a good medical checkup. Denise became alarmed and wanted to know why Mary was asking. Mary told her mother of her conversation with Bob the night before. She said there had been a lot written lately about depression, especially in older people, and it just seemed like a good idea for both of them to get thorough medical assessments from time to time, especially in light of the changes in her father's behaviour. Denise replied that both she and Al had had a good checkup two years ago but hadn't had any reason to see a doctor since, and that was a blessing.

Still, Mary urged her mother to arrange medical checkups for both of them. She reminded her that just as she, Bob, and the kids get annual checkups, so should her parents. And, Mary argued, it was a matter of something more than a regular routine examination, because it seemed clear that something was not right with her father, and the problem had to be identified and addressed.

Later that day Denise sat with Al on their deck, having a glass of wine before dinner. Al lately had started drinking more than a glass before dinner. He said it calmed him down, and Denise didn't think much about it. After all, they were retired, and he didn't have to worry about sleeping in if he had an extra drink or two.

She suggested that it was probably time for them both to go for a checkup; their doctor was still practising in Toronto, so they could make a day of it — see the doctor, do some shopping, and then come home. Al shot back that he didn't need a medical checkup; he felt just fine, and if she needed one, he'd be pleased to take her. He wouldn't explain why he refused to go, even though Denise asked several times. Finally, Al stated emphatically that he felt just fine, that there was no use spending time on something that wasn't necessary, and that Denise was probably fine, too. He said they were having the best years of their lives, and that's the way it should be. End of discussion. No matter what approach she took, Denise couldn't get Al to agree to visit the doctor.

A couple of days later, when Mary called to talk with her mother, Denise told her of her father's firm decision and said she didn't want to provoke him or have an argument about it. So, for the time being, Denise said, they would skip the visit to the doctor and just see how things went, because actually both of them felt well, other than the change in Al's interests and the fact that he seemed to sit around a lot more than usual. And after all, Denise told her daughter, there was really nothing physically wrong with them. Just because Al didn't want to build shelves or sail as often and wasn't that interested in sex, it didn't really mean anything. These things happen to people; she figured that it was a phase that would pass.

Mary didn't argue or push, feeling that she should respect her parents' wishes. For all her life, they'd been there for her as solid supporters and sound parents, and she didn't think the current situation demanded any kind of hard push on her part. She decided that if there were any further signs of a problem with her father, she'd personally arrange for and take him to a doctor's appointment. And her mother seemed just fine.

THE HEALTH CARE PROFESSIONAL'S POINT OF VIEW

It is imperative that Al get medical advice. It appears from the description that he is suffering from a depressive illness, which could be occurring for several reasons. Depressive symptoms can be the earliest manifestations of dementia, such as Alzheimer's disease, and major depression can occur for the first time in older individuals. Also, sometimes an earlier bout of depression may not have been recognized for what it was, or may have been attributed to nerves or stress or overwork, and therefore ignored and not formally treated. A family history of depression sometimes helps with the diagnosis, and it would be useful to know if any of Al's siblings or his parents ever had problems with mood disorders.

The main obstacle to Al's receiving help for depression is either that he is not aware something is wrong or, more likely, that he feels ashamed or guilty about admitting that things are not quite right. Many older people, especially men who have always been in charge, have difficulty admitting that things are happening to them that they cannot control. Deep-seated feelings of inadequacy often occur and sexual problems are not uncommon. This just makes things worse, especially if the person is not used to expressing feelings and exploring problems with other people, even his or her spouse.

The danger of depression, especially when it occurs in older men, is that it sometimes leads to suicide. They may not give any real outward warning that things are that bad, but to the surprise of their loved ones, they kill themselves, often by some violent means. Other men respond by withdrawing into themselves, eating less, or consuming increasing amounts of alcohol and medications such as tranquilizers (which they may get from a doctor after complaining of sleep problems) that temporarily ease their feelings of despair.

A family in this situation needs to find a way to get their loved one to see a physician. Some depressed people will go on their own so that they do not have to involve their family in a problem they may consider to be shameful. Some people believe that depression is a sign of weakness and that they should be able to just pull themselves out of it. But that rarely happens. So what are Mary and Denise to do? Waiting for something to happen is not the answer.

In fact, if they do that and something terrible happens they would never forgive themselves. It would probably be worthwhile for Mary and Denise to arrange to be alone with Al and have a discussion in which they express their concern for him because of what they have been observing for the past few months. Al's response may be dismissive and he may be angry that they are intruding on his feelings. It might be helpful for Mary to bring some reading material for Al, suggesting that he read it when he is alone. She and her mother have to express their love and devotion to Al and tell him that they realize just how difficult it might be for him to admit to or express his true feelings.

They might suggest that perhaps he would prefer to visit the doctor alone rather than going with Denise. Of course, the hope would be that he declines that offer, because they want to be with him when he tells the doctor what has been happening. By himself, he might deny that anything is wrong with his sense of self and value.

Al may not respond immediately to such a conversation. However, reading the material provided by Mary and Denise might persuade him to agree to see his doctor. If this is the case, it would be worthwhile communicating with the doctor first by phone or letter to explain the concerns of the family. Then, during the medical assessment, if Al does not admit to any problems, the physician can ask the necessary probing questions that may lead to a diagnosis of depression.

If a diagnosis of depression is made, the likely outcome will be an attempt at treatment with an antidepressant medication. There is a very good chance that the drug will be tolerated, especially if the physician begins with a small dose and gradually increases it, and will also be effective. If so, Al should become more sociable and less withdrawn and regain his interest in his hobbies and his wife. Many different antidepressant drugs and other components to treatment, including group therapy, may be offered, and usually one type of treatment or another will prove successful.

This is a time when a great deal of understanding and support is required, and Denise, Mary, and Bob will have to put all their efforts toward being supportive of Al and giving him the time and space to make his recovery.

One major concern, in addition to the high risk of suicide, is that the depression may be a symptom of dementia. For a substantial percentage of individuals, their depressive symptoms respond to treatment, but their mental powers and prowess continue to decline until it becomes clear that something beyond depression is taking place. The earliest signs of Alzheimer's disease are often revealed symptomatically with this kind of pattern. At present, there are no simple tests that can differentiate true late-onset depression from the type that will transform itself into dementia.

The positive news is that there are new drugs that many people with Alzheimer's disease appear to benefit from. Medical evidence suggests that even if there is no dramatic improvement in mental and cognitive function, the rate of progress of the disease appears to slow down, giving families and patients a bit more time to live life to its fullest and to make the necessary plans in anticipation of a progressive decline. (This includes taking steps such as appointing a power of attorney and making a will that will withstand external scrutiny or contest.) So, Mary and Denise need to lovingly get Al to the doctor, relate their observations, and explain their concerns. With a bit of luck, Al will be seen, a diagnosis of depression made, and proper treatment started. And maybe, with a little bit of extra luck, Al's condition will prove not to be the early stages of dementia.

Advancing Dementia:

When Life Gets More Difficult

When parents are deteriorating, their children must make some hard decisions about how they might best help them to be as secure and comfortable as possible, while trying to maintain their own lives and meeting their family commitments.

THE CHALLENGE

Dorothy Miller is an eighty-seven-year-old widow whose husband, Jack, died three years ago of lung cancer. Dorothy never got over the shock of his death, although Jack had a long period of painful illness. After Jack's funeral, Dorothy remained completely devastated and was often unable to stop crying for several hours at a time.

She continued to live in the one-bedroom apartment in a Moncton seniors' retirement home they'd moved to in the mid-1980s when Jack retired from his job with the railroad. They made the move partially to relieve the strain of caring for the house they had been living in and also because the seniors' facility offered increased levels of care. After Jack's death, Dorothy went out on her own less and less often and increasingly depended on her handful of friends who lived in the same building, as well as the staff, for personal services.

Although Dorothy was in relatively good physical condition when Jack died, shortly afterwards she began to have a number of complaints about her health. The physician who visited the seniors' home weekly saw Dorothy with increasing frequency. To help her sleep and to calm her nerves, he prescribed a mild dose of Lorazepam — a tranquilizer. Then, six months ago, Dorothy slipped in the lobby of the building, fell backwards, pulling her walker with her, and fractured one of her vertebrae. She was in a lot of pain and couldn't get up from the floor on her own. The nurse on duty was summoned and saw at once that Dorothy was suffering. The staff immediately called for an ambulance and she was taken to the hospital, where she required bedrest and fairly strong painkillers.

According to the doctor at the hospital, Dorothy became quite confused during the first night of her hospitalization, likely from a combination of codeine-containing pain medication and being in an unfamiliar place.

They kept her a few days longer to make sure she settled down, which she did. She was discharged and provided with some home care services, including a regimen of physiotherapy to help her get walking again.

Dorothy has one child, Owen, who lives in St. John's, Newfoundland. Owen is sixty-seven years old and has suffered from a degenerative disk condition for more than fifteen years; in fact, it's the reason he had to take early retirement from his job piloting fishing vessels. His wife, Louise, is three years his senior and for several decades has suffered from schizophrenia. Her illness is reasonably controlled by medications, but even so, she still has some very difficult times.

Owen and Louise chose to live in St. John's because Louise has supportive family there — two sisters and two brothers and their families, all of whom are very close to their sister. Also, Owen, who had always worked on or near the ocean, loves the sea and the city, and he is truly close to Louise's family. They have never had children.

While he has a deep sense of affection for his mother, he has never been terribly close to her, just as he hadn't been very close to his father. Owen has always respected his parents, but because he left home when he was eighteen years old and has lived away from Moncton since then, he simply never felt a pressing need to be physically close. In addition, neither parent had ever taken to Louise, and they never could accept that he'd married a "damaged woman," as his father had referred to her.

When Dorothy had her fall, the seniors' home called Owen to tell him what had happened and that his mother appeared to be all right, even though she had been admitted to hospital. Owen immediately travelled to Moncton to see his mother and spent three days there — the first while she was still in the hospital, and the other two back in her apartment.

Owen had seen his mother only once since his father's funeral, and he was surprised at how much she'd changed in three years. For one thing, Owen noticed how poorly his mother now moved; seldom would she even try to go from room to room without using at least a cane or, more often than not, her walker. He attributed this to her recent fall and painful back. Then he noticed that she often confused dates, times, and events. This alarmed him because he remembered that she had taken care of all her own banking since his father died, although there was never that much to do. When he asked his mother about her financial situation and if anyone was helping her with it, Dorothy told him that whenever she needs money, she calls someone at the bank who transfers the amount to her friend Wilma's account at the same bank, and then Wilma withdraws it and gives it to her. She also said that she writes only a few cheques and that her rent to the seniors' home was deducted automatically. Other than that, there wasn't much banking to be done.

During Owen's visit, he and his mother had dinner together in the main-floor dining room. Although Dorothy had some difficulty walking even with her walker as a result of the spinal compression fracture, she wanted to be where most of the residents took their meals.

During dinner Owen listened to his mother talk about some of the people she knew there. Even though she seemed to know something about most of them, she seemed to be vague about details. She also dropped veiled hints that perhaps some of the residents might be doing something wrong or, worse, illegal.

Owen spent most of his visit trying to arrange things for Dorothy so that she could maintain herself in the best possible way as she recovered from her injury. He requested some extra help in the room, including some bathing and dressing assistance. Dorothy initially declined this extra service, stating that she didn't need any help and that she didn't want anyone in her room for fear of having things stolen.

Over the course of his visit, Owen noted that he would have to repeat things he had told his mother over and over again because she kept forgetting what he'd said. But her memory for the "old days" was just fine, so he assumed that things could not be so bad if she could remember events from long ago in such detail. When he went home, other than the concern about his mother's memory problems, he was feeling that, all things considered, his mother was living safely and in relative comfort.

After his visit, Owen made sure he telephoned his mother once every two weeks for at least a few minutes. His conversations with her were relatively short, which didn't leave Dorothy much room to articulate in any detail any of her concerns or conditions. Owen didn't think he noticed any particular change in his mother, but he did sense that she acted as if he hadn't phoned before, and that she asked some of the same questions about himself and his life each time he called.

A few months after her accident, his mother did the totally unexpected — she called Owen. It was three o'clock in the morning and she wanted to know when his father was coming home, because she knew for a fact that he and Owen were at some party without her. Her voice was very tense, and when Owen said none of what she claimed was true, reminding her that Jack had been dead for years, Dorothy yelled at him to shut up and stop lying to her. Then she wanted to know how his "crazy wife" was, and Owen yelled back at his mother to stop talking like that and to listen. But she didn't. She just wanted to know over and over again when Jack would be back, and why Owen wouldn't help out and protect his aging, needy mother instead of going off to parties and living with some crazy woman.

By the time he got off the phone, Owen was devastated.

First thing in the morning he called the head of the seniors' home and talked to the administrator. What he heard floored Owen. The administrator said that ever since her fall Dorothy had been on a gradual slide in her state of health. She explained to Owen that there were a number of problems and that the doctor was concerned that his mother had signs of dementia, most likely Alzheimer's disease. She reported that Dorothy was still able to get to the dining room by herself and do her own grooming, although sometimes the mix and match of clothes was a bit out of character for her — but no one seemed to mind. And she was getting to the toilet on time, most of the time. But the administrator also told Owen that the staff was having someone help Dorothy with bathing all the time now, since she feels unsteady in the shower even though it has a chair in it to sit on.

The administrator suggested to Owen that he may want to try to visit more often and spend some time with his mother. She also reassured Owen that the seniors' home was equipped to care for people in Dorothy's situation, and that his mother was being moved to a floor where the staff could help residents with bathing, dressing, and, if necessary, preparing their food and sometimes even with feeding.

Owen then called the physician at the seniors' home. The doctor discussed some possible issues that might come up with Dorothy and suggested that Owen talk about them with his mother "before it was too late." Owen has never really discussed deep issues with his mother, having left home as a young adult. He wishes, now that his mother is failing and he finds himself unable to communicate with her in a more profound and personal manner, that he'd done more to develop his relationship with her over the years. However, he does know that his mother is not a religious person and stopped attending church many years ago, saying to him that there was not much in it for her. She had always seemed to be a practical person with no deep-seated sense of mystery or symbolism.

To Owen's surprise, when he did speak to his mother again, Dorothy was able to state quite emphatically that she would never want to be left to live as a "vegetable," should she get seriously ill. She seemed able to articulate clearly her wish that if her condition couldn't be treated easily and the prognosis was that she couldn't return to her present state of physical or mental health, Owen should "let her go from this world." Owen was quite relieved to hear Dorothy state things so clearly. The doctor reassured Owen that should Dorothy fall ill, her wishes for minimal intervention of high-technology medicine would be respected.

Owen told the doctor that he could be contacted in an emergency but that he trusted the physician's understanding of Dorothy's wishes should she be unable to express them at the time of a real medical crisis.

After these long-distance conversations, sitting in his small family room at the back of his frame house, Owen didn't know what else to do. He had his own personal challenges to face and suddenly he had an added responsibility to manage. He knows that Dorothy is safe for the time being, and he remains hopeful that he can provide sufficient support without having to leave home too often, because that is a physical, mental, and financial strain for him.

THE HEALTH CARE PROFESSIONAL'S POINT OF VIEW

The first thing Owen must do is figure out what has happened to Dorothy. It appears that she is suffering from some form of dementia, such as Alzheimer's disease, and perhaps something else as well. It is likely that she has been suffering from that condition for as long as a year prior to her fall. It does not seem likely that the fall itself caused her decline in mental function, but it is not uncommon for an acute medical event to lead to the recognition of dementia, which a person may have managed in his or her own environment for quite a while.

People with a moderate degree of dementia often succeed in managing their daily activities if they live in a reasonably supportive environment, such as a retirement home or seniors' building like the one in which Dorothy has been living. In Dorothy's case, for example, the staff at the bank have been very helpful, making sure that all of her financial transactions were conducted appropriately.

With a trauma like a fall, even if there is no head injury, which could potentially lead to a more rapid decline in mental function, the resultant hospitalization and need for analgesics containing codeine can increase the risk of a state of acute confusion, often referred to as delirium. This appears to be what happened to Dorothy. Although she made a reasonable recovery, the fact that the staff at the seniors' home has recommended an increased level of personal care assistance is an indication that her mental abilities are deteriorating.

If Owen were able to arrange it, Dorothy might benefit from a referral to a specialist in geriatrics, geriatric psychiatry, or neurology — someone who has a lot of experience with older adults, especially those who have complex medical conditions and problems related to dementia. One goal would be to differentiate the possible causes of her dementia in order to take the best available steps to deal with the condition and the possible consequences of it. Also, the specialist physician can act as one of the resource people Owen could to turn to should his mother experience further decline.

By reviewing the events leading to the present state of affairs (the "history"), considering the physical findings, and running some tests (possibly a CT scan or other brain imaging techniques and some blood tests), a physician may be better able to define the kind of dementia that has affected Dorothy. This process is important because age alone is not considered a basis for a decline in mental function such as Dorothy is experiencing.

Although the likelihood of dementia increases substantially as one ages, it is still important to try to define all the possible confounding causes of the particular condition. For example, it is possible that the fall Dorothy experienced was caused by a small stroke that also accentuated her apparently rapid mental decline. It may be that she has blood pressure problems that were not noted previously or problems with her cholesterol. When all the findings are put together, the physician might be in a position to recommend treatments that could be useful in dealing with underlying risk factors that could cause further unwanted events.

If the physician believes that Dorothy is suffering from Alzheimer's disease, it may be worthwhile to try one of the new medications available for this condition. Although they have been in use for only a few years, the evidence suggests that for a reasonable percentage of patients with Alzheimer's-type dementia (and those with some variants of that condition), these drugs can improve the level of mental awareness and interactions with people. In addition, it appears that the drugs decrease the rate of further decline of the condition, thereby keeping patients in a more stable condition for a longer period of time.

Dorothy may respond to the medication, which could improve the way she functions. But she may not respond, and decline may continue despite any medical treatments. Dorothy could potentially become more agitated, and the paranoia that Owen witnessed during that disturbing telephone call may become more apparent and interfere with her ability to function well in the social environment of the home in which she is presently living.

The next question Owen has to face is where his mother will live as her condition deteriorates. The seniors' home claims it can provide a level of care called "assisted living," but should Dorothy need greater care than the facility and its staff can provide, she would have to move to a nursing home. It would be worthwhile for Owen to visit some of the nursing homes in the vicinity and speak to the staff at Dorothy's home to find out what their experiences have been with the homes in the region. He should understand the process so he knows when to register her for admission, assuming there is a waiting list for some of the homes that he and Dorothy like. Owen needs to set his mother up in a reasonably safe and secure environment that will be able to handle the likely decline in her condition, especially since he lives so far away.

To make the best choice, Owen should discuss with the administrator of the home, as well as her family physician, all aspects of Dorothy's physical needs and stress that he wants his mother's stated wishes to be respected as she declines.

Visiting his mother is difficult for Owen, but he could arrange to speak to the nurse at the seniors' home once a week, just to catch up on things. He should also continue to call his mother, of course, and could establish a routine of always phoning on the same day at the same time so that his mother is more likely to remember. It would help put Owen's mind at ease if he could also arrange for a friend or neighbour in the seniors' residence to keep an eye out for Dorothy and to call Owen if there were ever any worries.

Like so many children who live far away from ailing parents, Owen has to cope as well as he can. All he can do — all anyone can do — is try to do the best job possible.

WE'RE ON OUR OWN:

How to Plan for the Future

A couple in their mid-sixties must consider how long and effectively they can care for an aging mother while planning for the day they will retire and eventually require care themselves.

THE CHALLENGE

Jean and Frank Scott have lived on the outskirts of Peterborough, Ontario, for more than thirty years, after having moved from Kingston where they were both born, raised, and educated. Jean is sixty-two and Frank is sixty-five. Jean is a schoolteacher and plans to work until she retires at sixty-five because she loves her job and the kids, and also because she wants to maximize her retirement pension. Frank runs the local hardware store. It has been a touch-and-go affair over the years, but it does have some value, and Frank hopes to keep the store going and then, when the time is right, sell it and make some profit from the capital that's been invested in it. Jean and Frank also have some RRSPs and various modest investments that they have been making to save for their retirement.

They have many friends and neighbours in the surrounding area but no children of their own. Jean has a sister who lives in Newfoundland with her family, and Frank has a brother and sister who still live in Kingston with their families. Jean's mother, Louise, aged eighty-seven, has lived with Jean and Frank since she lost her husband eight years ago. Her income is limited to little more than her OAS (Old Age Security) and GIS (Guaranteed Income Supplement).

Louise managed well until about a year ago when she fell and broke her hip and had some complications, including a stroke that was either caused by the fall or happened just after it. She was found to have an irregular heartbeat and has since required Coumadin (a blood thinner). She is also a long-standing diabetic and for the past few years has required insulin injections.

Although Louise has made a good recovery from the fracture and the stroke, she hasn't really been the same since and can't help much around the house. In fact, she now needs help with several normal personal activities. Because Jean and Frank both work, and there is no other family nearby, they've been dependent on the Ontario home care system to help provide in-home support for Louise, including bathing and meal assistance and helping her with insulin injections and monitoring her blood sugar. Because Jean can get home from school by about four o'clock on the days she doesn't have after-school meetings and Frank has some flexibility with the store when he has adequate help, they've managed with these limited care services provided through the local Community Care Access Centre (CCAC).

Early last fall, Frank and Jean received notice that the hours allotted to Louise's care were to be cut substantially because of funding restrictions to the CCAC by the provincial government. As a result, they've had to make some private arrangements with neighbours, friends, and a number of local teenagers to fill in the gaps left by the reductions. They are paying for the assistance, but their real concern is not the financial drain; it is the prospect of what will happen should Louise require more care. It will be a real challenge to make sure that she gets the services she needs without putting enormous pressure on Jean and Frank. They worry that they won't be able to afford to keep Louise at home should she deteriorate to the point that she requires full-time help. Moreover, they've been thinking about what will happen to them during the next number of years should they fall ill themselves and need social services. Since they don't have any children or other family in the vicinity, they've expressed these concerns to their physician and the social worker from the CCAC who worked with them in providing care for Louise. They're feeling very vulnerable in terms of their ability to cope with Louise's needs, physically and financially, and at risk in terms of their own future.

THE HEALTH CARE PROFESSIONAL'S POINT OF VIEW

There are two main issues involved here, the first being the very real and immediate anxiety about how to provide Louise with the best care possible while not putting Frank and Jean at emotional and financial risk. It is necessary for them both to continue working to maintain their income for as long as possible, as their retirement pensions and savings are not sufficient to assure them a reasonably comfortable retirement for themselves, much less to ensure that Louise's needs will be met in the future.

They should have a very frank discussion with Louise about the issues and options and let her know that they will do whatever they can to continue to look after her. But they must also tell her that if circumstances change and they cannot continue with this plan, they will look for a nursing home that is close by and suitable for her. They should make it clear that this plan is not meant to abandon Louise, but rather to make sure that they can continue to participate in looking after her and still preserve their energy.

The financial implications may vary depending on Louise's income, but if she does not have anything beyond her OAS and GIS, there should be no other funding expected from Frank and Jean for her nursing home care. They would clearly take all the necessary steps to make sure the facility is the one most suited to her needs, and it is obvious from their history and relationship that they would visit her frequently and take part in as many social activities as possible, including taking her home for weekends and holidays whenever they could.

The second issue, Jean and Frank's concern about their own future, is more difficult to address. The future is always impossible to predict. Government policies could change so that society may become more senior-friendly. Access to necessary health care and social services may not be a major problem. Or, of course, the opposite could become the case and those without supportive families or friends may be in deep trouble should things go wrong in terms of health or independence. What Jean and Frank can do, at least, is discuss their concerns with the family that they do have — their siblings and nieces or nephews — so that should they fall ill and need some support, their preferences are known.

Preparing a living will, with the assistance of their physician, may help them feel comfortable with some of the difficult decisions that might be necessary in the future. Just naming a relative or close friend to be a surrogate decision-maker and making clear their hopes and expectations for a time when they can't make decisions for themselves could lessen their worries. If they are not sure they can count on anyone, they can turn to their lawyer and ask him or her to take on the role. In retirement homes or seniors' residences, should they eventually move into one, there is usually a way to get someone to agree to act as a support person or surrogate should the situation require it.

So, although it is understandable for them to feel some anxiety, especially as they face Louise's decline and the extra demands made on them, Frank and Jean can take many steps to assure themselves of safe and secure later years.

If the time comes when they are no longer able to look after Louise, Frank and Jean have to examine the options for her long-term care, and there are many considerations. When looking for a long-term care facility, the options are often limited by geography. In some smaller communities there may be only one facility close by, and depending on the jurisdiction that facility may range from a retirement home with or without an assisted-living level of care to a regulated long-term care facility. Retirement homes usually fall under the category of unregulated homes because in most jurisdictions governments do not provide a regulatory framework under which such facilities function.

Some of the better homes of this nature belong to voluntary organizations that try to ensure some reasonable level of quality of care — but staffing levels and services are not mandated by government. The facilities are usually privately run, sometimes as part of provincial or national chains. In some the quality of care is very high and the services personalized, but the cost, too, may be very high, and there is usually no subsidy offered by government. Many retirement homes, especially those with assisted-living levels of care, provide services that in other situations are usually carried out by long-term care facilities, often known as nursing homes or homes for the aged.

In some jurisdictions there is a range of options within a framework of special care housing structures that also provide important and supportive care. There are various kinds of group homes for those with physical and/or psycho-social problems. Many facilities of this sort provide excellent care for individuals with special kinds of problems, such as dementia of the Alzheimer's type.

When the option exists, many families try to get their loved one admitted to a regulated long-term care facility because the provincial government covers some of the costs and regulates the standard of care. The facilities themselves may be under the control of private for-profit corporations, government (usually municipal), or not-for-profit organizations.

The last category often includes community organizations, religious, cultural or ethnic organizations, or those related to some common heritage or historical link. (These facilities are sometimes referred to as "charitable homes for the aged.") Many large cities have long-term care facilities that reflect the ethnic and cultural bias of that community. For example, in Toronto there are Catholic, Muslim, and Jewish homes for the aged as well as those that cater to the Chinese, Italian, Greek, Finnish, and Polish communities — to name just a few.

The attraction of the not-for-profit facilities is the assumption that there is a source of commitment to the care of the elderly beyond that of financial profit. The standards of care and dedication may be better than those run by private companies that may be accountable to share-holders and other corporate interests. Having said that, there are certainly many for-profit organizations, some of which belong to large chains, that provide excellent service and quality care.

Probably the two most important considerations when choosing a long-term care facility are location and quality of care. Ideally the facility should be convenient to family members to enable them to visit easily, so that frequent short visits can take place, which are preferable to infrequent but longer visits.

Of course, the quality of care is paramount but can be difficult to assess. One worthwhile exercise is to ask other people who have loved ones living in the facility what they think. You can also ask if there has been an accreditation process and whether the facility has received accreditation or if you can access recent inspection reports. Of course, a visit to the facility to watch how residents are treated and the sense of pride that the staff demonstrate in what they are doing can give a pretty good idea about the standards of care and caring. However, sometimes quality of care can only be assessed after the fact, so close observation during the acclimatization process is crucial. How is your loved one progressing? How often do the staff meet with families? How accessible are they? Answering these questions may indicate the quality of care that is being provided.

When you move a loved one into a long-term care facility, it is worth finding out who's who in the staff hierarchy and who should be contacted for information and progress. Providing the staff with health care expectations is very useful. For example, if a living will exists, the staff should be provided with a copy, or at least be told of the person's wishes for treatment and care. A meeting with the assigned or chosen physician (depending on the situation) is useful to make sure that both you and the doctor understand the general goals of care and the parameters around which medical care will be provided.

Some individuals are too frail and sick to be cared for in long-term care facilities. For example, individuals who require tube feeding or a respirator or complete bowel and bladder care or who are bedridden or semi-conscious may need to be in a chronic-care hospital, which has a different framework of care than what is provided in long-term care facilities. Admission to such a hospital-type facility is usually based on a medical decision and may be as the family's first choice or as a transfer from a long-term care facility, should the person's condition deteriorate to the point that care can no longer be safely provided in the long-term care facility.

Choosing the right facility is very difficult for a family, and sometimes the bureaucratic process can be daunting to even the most informed. The decision-making process often seems very rushed to families struggling emotionally with the decisions. If possible, family members should seek the advice and assistance of a social worker who is knowledgeable in the field and familiar with the peculiar needs and preferences of the family. But the difficult decisions have to be made, and whatever those decisions are, the challenge is to make the best of it by being a loving and supportive family member and exploring ways to help the staff and the facility fulfill their goals to the best of their professional and organizational ability.

You may have the chance to join a family council or advisory group or volunteer to participate in recreational programs to augment the care and programs provided by the staff. Positive and engaged participation is usually far more productive and results in a better sense of dedication from the staff than constant complaining and finding fault, which unfortunately is the way that some families approach long-term care facilities. Constructive criticism is usually well received by a reputable organization, but more effective than criticism is a positive and participatory attitude from the loving family members who help those directly in the caregiving role.

Caring is infectious, and staff usually recognize family members who truly care for their loved ones, and they usually respond in a positive fashion that helps everyone.

FINDING A NEW LIFE:

Corrections and Concerns

Many elderly people who have lost a spouse want to move forward and "get a life" at some point, yet often their children find themselves unable to understand or approve. This inevitably leads to confusion and potential conflict.

THE CHALLENGE

When Don Benson died after a lingering illness, his wife, Nora, understandably grieved for more than a year and a half. They'd been married for fifty-one years, and it had been a happy marriage throughout. They'd been extremely close — not just as husband and wife and parents, but as the closest of friends and confidants. In fact, while they'd had many friends and a very active social life, they always told everyone that the best free time was the time they spent alone together.

Nora found much comfort and solace in the support she got from her son, Jeremy, and daughter, Lisa, at the time of Don's death. They stayed very close to her for the first few months and, even after, kept a close watch over her. They visited and phoned frequently and brought her to their homes.

Some six months after the funeral, Nora told her children that she appreciated their kindness, but she was feeling more stable and wanted some time to herself — to think about her life with Don, to sort things in the house, and to reflect. While Jeremy and Lisa at first worried that their mother was sliding into some kind of depression, they discovered, much to their relief, that she seemed to be all right being more on her own.

At the time of Don's death, Nora was still a relatively young senior citizen of seventy-two years. She was in good health; the only significant medical procedure she'd had was cataract surgery three years earlier.

Jeremy was forty-four years old and working long hours as a fairly successful stock broker when his father died. He was married to Espeth, a very happy woman who worked part-time at an upscale clothing boutique and spent as much time as possible with their eleven-year-old daughter, Dawn.

His sister, Lisa, had just turned forty. She lived in a common-law relationship with Marvin. They had no children, and they always explained that they'd never intended to have a family because both were devoted to their careers and each other. Lisa was an actress who regularly landed supporting roles in local playhouse productions and appeared in television commercials and print ads. Marvin was a graphic artist by day and an aspiring painter by night, working on canvases that were displayed in some smaller galleries and in various restaurants.

The two families got along well, despite being very different. And both really wanted to help Nora in any way they could.

During the period Nora wanted to spend more time alone, her children and their families pulled back, respecting her wish. Of course, they still visited her and invited her to visit them and they all spent time together during holidays and birthdays and other special events. Jeremy and Lisa also each spoke to their mother on the phone a couple of times a week.

As time passed, Nora seemed to regain her sense of confidence in herself and in life in general. She spoke less of the "good times with

Don" and more about how she was going to move into a retirement home in the next year or so, about the canasta card club she'd joined, about her church activities, and about a local book club that she was thinking of joining. She also announced plans to become a volunteer at the local museum, a place that she has always enjoyed.

Her children were amazed and thrilled at what they considered to be a very healthy approach by their mother to the rest of her life. They were also delighted that Nora looked good; she dressed well, moved with comfort, and spoke clearly and lucidly about her life and day-to-day activities.

Six months ago, Nora told her children that she'd selected a retirement home and planned to sell the family home and move out within the year. She also surprised them with the news that she was going to take a seniors' bus tour across Canada that would last three weeks. She'd already signed up for the tour, which was departing a week after her announcement. Jeremy and Lisa asked their mother if she thought that was wise. Nora assured them it was perfectly safe and told them with some pride that she'd had her annual medical checkup recently and had been given a clean bill of health. She also reminded them how much she and Don used to enjoy going on bus tours and train rides and cruises.

And so Nora headed off, promising not to just send post cards, but to call either Jeremy or Lisa every few days. She did just that, and she always sounded cheerful and contented. The three weeks seemed a long time to her children, who worried about her since she'd never been on any trip alone before.

But Nora returned unscathed and unharmed. If anything, at the "welcome back" dinner they arranged for her she seemed brighter and happier than they'd seen her in a long time. It was during the dinner that Nora told her children and their spouses that her life had changed. She explained that a few months earlier she'd met a very nice widower named Albert at the canasta club. He was seventy-six years old, tall, very considerate, and fun to be with. They'd had dinner together a few times. He was the one who suggested she go on the tour, for which he had already signed up, and they'd just spent a lot of time together and were very comfortable with each other. He, too, liked reading and had joined the book club and thought that the museum volunteer activity was great fun. And he lived at the retirement home where she planned to move.

Jeremy and Lisa were flabbergasted, as were Espeth and Marvin. They had not expected this at all. They didn't know what to say as they exchanged glances across the dinner table. It was only when Nora asked what they thought that they each said it was a surprise.

Jeremy immediately wanted to know more about Albert — about his health, about his financial situation, about his family. He had a lot of questions that just bubbled out of him. Lisa remained very quiet and listened to her mother patiently talk about her new friend.

After Jeremy had taken Nora home, he called Lisa. They talked for quite a while and agreed that this wasn't like their mother. They just couldn't imagine her finding someone else at this stage in her life. It simply didn't feel right to them, especially since their mother and father had been so close. Jeremy pointed out that he'd heard a lot of stories about widows and widowers who had hit on other elderly people in order to ensure their own comfort and financial security. He told her stories of stocks being transferred to such people in good faith, only to be cashed in by that trusted person who then vanishes. It was an unsettling phone conversation for them both.

Lisa had yet another nagging concern, and she called her mother the next day to raise it. Lisa asked her mother how she really felt about this man; Lisa wasn't comfortable calling him by his name. Her mother responded that she felt very comfortable and wanted to know why her daughter was asking. Lisa finally said what was bothering her: she loved her father and her memories of him, and of her father and mother together, and she just couldn't see how Nora could toss all that aside and select another man.

Nora was stunned and hurt. She told her daughter that one had nothing to do with the other. She said that tears still came to her eyes and she felt an ache in her heart when she thought about Don, but there was nothing she could do to bring him back; she could only cling to the good memories. But, she reminded Lisa, she still had a life and she wanted to live it. Besides, she and Albert were just friends, nothing more.

That didn't satisfy Lisa, and they ended the conversation on a tense note. Later, Lisa called Jeremy and reported what their mother had told her. Neither felt good about the developments, but nor did they know what to do about it. The only decision they made was that together they must convince their mother to abandon her friendship with Albert.

A few days later Jeremy and Lisa went to see their mother to talk about their concerns. Nora became agitated and defensive and asked her children to let her have a life she could enjoy. They ended the session in a standoff — Nora determined to carry on with her plans, and Jeremy and Lisa equally determined to change her mind.

THE HEALTH CARE PROFESSIONAL'S POINT OF VIEW

The death of a spouse often leads children to assume that the surviving parent will remain single and that their role as children will be to care for and nurture the parent as a single widow or widower.

In many cultures the idea of remarriage is quite alien, and widows especially bear the mark of their status quite openly. It is unusual for them to reconnect for many reasons, including societal standards and family expectations. But in other cultures it is considered terrible for someone to be alone after the death of a spouse, and a lot of effort goes into trying to reconnect the person (especially in the case of widowers; the gender bias is clear).

In Canada and the rest of North America it is not uncommon for widows and widowers to remarry, although the likelihood for men is much greater than for women simply because there are many more older women than men. Also, our cultural bias finds it more acceptable for men to connect with much younger women than for women to take up with younger men.

So what's the problem with Nora's family? One would have thought they would be delighted that their mother is in a position to have a meaningful relationship at this time of her life. But it is not uncommon for children to react exactly as Jeremy and Lisa have. It would be useful for Jeremy and Lisa to explore the cause of their reaction so that they can come to understand it and prevent undermining their relationship with Nora or alienating her and her newfound "friend," who may someday become more of a "significant other."

Children often have emotional reactions to situations without looking at the situation from the perspective of the most important person affected by the situation, who in this case is Nora. Jeremy and Lisa seem to be forgetting that Nora's needs and wishes should be paramount, and as much as possible they should be supporting her to be a physically and emotionally independent person. If they really thought about it, they would probably come to the conclusion that if either of them were struck by the tragedy of losing a spouse, they too might one day want to reconnect. Emotional and physical relationships are so central to human happiness and fulfillment that to deny people such opportunities is to condemn them to a life of loneliness.

A lot of children think of a parent's desire to reconnect as somehow compromising the respect and love for the deceased spouse. Yet if you ask those in loving relationships what they would want for their spouse if they died, most would say that the most important thing would be that their loved one not be left alone and that they should try to find someone else with whom to share an emotional and physical relationship.

Some children are repelled by the thought that their parent might actually want to have a sexual relationship with another person, especially when they are older and after so many years with their other parent. Many younger people erroneously assume that human sexuality stops at a certain age. In fact the main barrier to healthy and fulfilling sexual relationships in the older years is the lack of a partner rather than the lack of desire or physical ability.

Lastly, there may be other concerns that the children are not expressing that are financial in nature. Sometimes a surviving parent is left with a lot of money and assets that the children assume will pass to them after the death of the surviving spouse. Therefore, a potential new spouse can be seen as a threat to an inheritance. It is also true that sometimes dishonest individuals prey on unsuspecting widows and widowers to take advantage of their financial situation, using their emotional relationship as the basis for poor financial decision-making. I have seen very few of these cases in my practice of more than twenty-five years, but indeed this might be a valid concern of children who want to be sure not only of their future inheritance but also of the financial security of the surviving parent.

So what should the children do? Presumably they want to continue to have a loving relationship with their mother and at the same time ensure their mother's happiness and their collective financial security. If they keep acting the way they are, they are not going to achieve their goals.

The first step is for them to sit down with Nora and express to her their support and happiness that she is finding her own life again and that they respect and love her for it. They should also say that they understand why it is so important that she find a potential partner for an emotional and, possibly, a physical relationship. They must emphasize their support for her happiness as a major priority in their lives.

With that said, they can then say that they just want to be sure that this new relationship does not put Nora at any risk, emotionally, physically, or financially. They should offer to meet Albert and arrange a time when they can do so in a relaxed manner and welcome him as a special person in their mother's life The more they include him in family events, the more likely they will be able to figure out what kind of person he is and how he and Nora seem together.

With that kind of approach Jeremy and Lisa will be in a much better position to express other opinions and concerns. For example, they might suggest that should the relationship develop into something more serious or legally binding, Nora should seek the advice of a lawyer to make sure that her financial resources are protected. In addition, if Nora wants to protect her children's financial inheritance, there are legal ways of doing so. Taking such a step would probably go a long way in soothing the suspicions and concerns that the children might rightfully have but may not be able to articulate to themselves or to Nora as they contend with this new situation.

Many older people reconnect very successfully in their later years, especially after the loss of a long-time spouse. What more wonderful thing could happen to people who would otherwise spend their remaining years dependent on their children and friends? A new partner does not desecrate the honour of the previous spouse; if anything, many people who have been through such experiences find that they can share the importance of the previous relationship and use it as a basis for a new and fulfilling relationship. Children can play an important role in supporting and encouraging their parents' independence and need for emotional and physical fulfillment — an essential part of human existence.

DECISION TIME:

Planning for the Inevitable

When one parent is ill and the other parent appears to be unable to make appropriate caregiving choices, the children must make some hard decisions about what steps to take to protect the dignity and well-being of both.

THE CHALLENGE

Margit and Tamas Ujhazy were childhood sweethearts. They were born in the same small village in Hungary, and they married when she was sixteen and he was nineteen. A few years later, they immigrated to Saskatchewan when Canada was encouraging people to come to work in this country. Under the terms of the agreement with the government, for the first five years they had to work on a farm — which is what they did back in their native Hungary. After the five-year period expired, they moved to Esterhazy, where they rented a room in a private home and worked in the area — he as a farmhand, and she as a domestic.

They never prospered but lived frugally, and when Margit was expecting their first child they bought a tiny four-room bungalow that has been their home since the late-1950s.

Now, Margit is seventy and Tamas is seventy-three. Margit had a serious stroke a year ago that has left her totally incapacitated and in need of round-the-clock care in a nursing home. She is able to speak, but not easily, and often mixes English with Hungarian. Meanwhile, Tamas continues to live in their home and work part-time at a local hardware store.

They have two children — Elizabeth, forty, and Arpad, thirty-seven. Elizabeth, a radiologist, lives in Vancouver with her second husband, Bob, a software programmer. Arpad, a chartered accountant with a consulting firm, lives in Edmonton with his wife, Nancy, and their three children. Since leaving home, neither Elizabeth nor Arpad had been very close to each other or to their parents, until their mother's stroke prompted both siblings to become more actively involved.

When their mother suffered her stroke, Tamas called his children — something he hadn't done in more than a decade — to tell them what had happened. Both Elizabeth and Arpad went to Esterhazy to see their mother and visit with their father. It was Elizabeth's first visit home in more than five years and Arpad's first time back home in four years. Elizabeth and Arpad now call their father every Sunday and stay in touch with each other through weekly emails to compare notes about what Tamas has told them.

Recently, their mother was diagnosed with bone cancer. Tamas told them about the diagnosis in one of their weekly telephone calls but said that everything was under control. In a subsequent telephone conversation he told Elizabeth that nursing home staff had complained that Margit yells a lot and said that they think that she's in extreme pain. But Tamas says she's not really in much pain at all; rather, all the noise she's making and the claims of pain are her way to get more attention.

Elizabeth asks her father who their family doctor is and decides to call her. When they eventually connect, the doctor tells Elizabeth that Margit is indeed in extreme pain, which is why she's often yelling out.

The doctor wants to place her on morphine patches but explains that Tamas refuses to agree and, at most, allows only Tylenol #3 to be administered. The doctor also tells Elizabeth that Tamas, who's been diagnosed with early signs of Alzheimer's, proudly points out that his wife has a history of bearing pain very well. Tamas has said that while everything possible should be done to keep Margit alive, morphine patches are unacceptable. It's not clear to the doctor why Tamas feels that way.

Now Elizabeth and Arpad face a dilemma. The doctor has explained Tamas's wishes and suggested that their father may not be making choices in a sound frame of mind. Elizabeth and Arpad agree that Arpad should see their father to talk about what needs to be done for both their parents. Uncertain of what they should do about either parent, the two siblings decide that their father's views should be sought and, if they make sense, applied.

When Arpad meets his father in Esterhazy, Tamas tells him that his mother often took to yelling out loud when she felt she was in pain but that this was a natural overreaction that shouldn't be taken seriously. He reminds Arpad how much and how loud Margit used to yell even if she just bumped an elbow into a door or got a slight cut on a finger. Arpad can't remember any yelling at all by his mother, so while he wants to believe his father, he's very conscious that his mother is suffering terribly from her bone cancer while incapacitated by her stroke.

No matter how much he talks to his father during his weekend visit, Arpad can't convince him to approve the morphine patches or any other pain management assistance for his mother. And the more they talk, the more Arpad realizes that at times his father is very logical and lucid, but at other times he is seemingly confused and uncertain of past events. Arpad wants to believe his father, yet he's torn by nagging doubts and a growing concern for his mother's condition. By the end of the weekend, Arpad feels the visit was an exercise in futility and that even if his mother has a low pain threshold, that has nothing to do with the fact that she has bone cancer, which he recalls is one of the most painful types of cancer there is.

When Arpad returns home, he calls his sister and they have a long discussion about what they can and should do for both their parents. Both realize that there is little they can do long-distance and that neither really wants to take on the responsibility of becoming a dedicated family caregiver. They exchange stories of their childhood and teenage years that demonstrate that their parents didn't do as much as they should have for either of them — and then they realize that they are groping for a justification to do little or nothing.

Ashamed, agitated, and confused, Elizabeth and Arpad finally decide that they must try to help make their mother's suffering as manageable as possible and that they need to try to deal with their father and find a way to get him the help he'll need when their mother dies and as his Alzheimer's continues to develop.

The Health Care Professional's Point of View

Elizabeth and Arpad face a situation in which there really isn't a right answer. Here they have one parent who appears to be suffering unnecessarily from pain due to cancer and another whose dignity they are trying to respect, even as he shows evidence of cognitive decline. The respect for one parent's needs appears to be in direct conflict with the needs of the other parent. As both children try to show respect for their parents, they must struggle with the impact of whatever decision they make.

To ignore the need for proper pain management in a parent suffering from malignant bone pain seems cruel and unacceptable to them. However, since their father is the person making decisions, they are trying to respect him even though the consequences for their mother are not acceptable emotionally, nor are they acceptable as part of a standard of medical practice for palliative care.

Most health care professionals consider withholding pain control in the palliative stage of malignant disease to be an abrogation of one's professional responsibility. Therefore, in order to care for their mother and try to maintain respect for their father, Elizabeth and Arpad are going to require enormous sympathy and assistance from the health care professionals caring for both of their parents.

If, indeed, Tamas is showing early evidence of Alzheimer's, this should be formally addressed by his physician. It might be that the diagnosis is incorrect and that there is another explanation for the change in his personality and decision-making process. For example, depression can appear to cause memory lapses and other cognitive changes that may be misdiagnosed as dementia of the Alzheimer's type. Some medications (such as sleeping pills and sedatives) can also cause lapses in cognition, memory, and judgment, and Tamas's doctor should evaluate this possibility in an objective fashion.

If, after appropriate review, assuming that Tamas agrees to the evaluation (which can be facilitated by his physician if the children explain the situation), no clear clinical explanation for his views and no disorder that might compromise his ability to be a surrogate decision-maker is found, the children are faced with a serious problem. They will have to get as much assistance as possible from physicians and nurses whom their father trusts to try to help him understand the importance of proper pain management for their mother. It would be worth exploring why he is opposed to morphine patches. If he is concerned about her becoming addicted or overly somnolent, perhaps alternative methods of pain management might be suggested that he will not perceive as risky or that might "end Margit's life." This might include a less potent analgesic given on a round-the-clock basis coupled with drugs such as tricylclic antidepressants that can accentuate the effects of analgesics.

If Tamas still refuses some appropriate regimen of pain management, the children will have to decide whether they should apply to replace their father as surrogate decision-maker because of his failure to fulfill this role according to most legal frameworks (i.e., acting in the best interests of the person on whose behalf you are acting). This will not be an easy decision and could potentially cause a rift, temporary or otherwise, in the relationship between Elizabeth and Arpad and their father.

If, on the other hand, it is found clinically that their father is cognitively impaired and incapable of making proper surrogate decisions, he can be replaced by the children. This may also result in a negative response from him, the only difference being that the children can

perhaps get some help from the physician in explaining why the sur-
rogacy has to be changed. In that way, the doctor can bear some of the
responsibility for the decision, and then proper decisions concerning
Margit's palliative needs can be made without the children appearing
to be going against the wishes of their father.

The children must be prepared for the likelihood that after their
mother dies, their father is going to require an extra measure of help. If
he is, indeed, manifesting evidence of dementia and early Alzheimer's,
he may feel the loss of his wife profoundly and his symptoms may be
exaggerated. It is likely that he will need help in his home. Or perhaps
he will eventually need to live elsewhere. Such a decision should not be
taken precipitously, but rather in a measured manner, as the mourning
period may be prolonged.

The hope is that their father's dignity can be maintained as much as
possible while they still meet the first imperative — ensuring that their
mother has a peaceful and pain-free death.

END OF LIFE:

Caring and Sharing

It's natural for children to become intensely concerned and involved when a parent is in the process of dying, and even more so when the other parent isn't well. The real challenge is to know how to become constructively involved rather than intrusive.

THE CHALLENGE

Simon Delacroix is seventy-three years old and dying of lung cancer. His wife, Emma, is the same age. Because she's a severe diabetic and more than forty pounds overweight, as well as physically and mentally exhausted from trying to care for her husband over the past two years, Emma is no longer able to care for Simon with the level of intensity required.

They live in Windsor, Ontario, in their three-bedroom suburban home. They have regular help with lawn and snow care. As Simon's condition continues to deteriorate and Emma is ever less capable of caring for him in their home, they've turned to the local Community Care Access Centre (CCAC) for additional support. With budgetary constraints, that support is nominal — a homemaker who comes to help bathe Simon and do some light housecleaning twice a week for two hours each visit.

Simon and Emma have one child, Allison, who is forty-six years old. She lives in London, Ontario — a bit less than a two-hour drive away — with her husband, Daryl, and their two children, Melissa and Mary. Allison works as a bank teller, and Daryl is a program director with the city's parks and recreation department. Allison has tried to help her parents as best she can, but Simon and Emma have been stubborn all along, consistently rejecting her repeated pleas to have her father put in a nursing home so he can get the attention and services he needs and to reduce the pressure on her mother.

Simon, Emma, Allison, and her husband are fully cognizant that, according to their family doctor and the oncologist who's been examining him, Simon will probably die within the next four to six months. However, the family is having a very difficult — nearly impossible — time talking about it in any constructive fashion. They're frozen in inaction.

Simon is in a state of denial. He rationalizes his terminal condition and most days proclaims that "this is the first day of the rest of my life, and I'm going to improve." While this may seem a positive mental attitude, with Simon it's actually a deep longing to regain his health while wishing away the reality of the situation.

Emma, meanwhile, is angry that Simon didn't stop smoking years ago when she did. She blames him for being on the verge of a premature death, and while trying to make him as comfortable as possible, she too often verbally attacks him for his selfishness and lack of self-control. Emma is emotionally distraught, and she is also worried about her own health, placing the blame directly on her husband for the state of their lives.

And instead of appreciating Allison's concerns and expressions of support, both parents blame their daughter for meddling in what they believe is their own problem. They can't see her as the adult she is. Allison, in their minds, is still a child who should listen to their words and wisdom and show respect for their wishes, which are entrenched in a paradigm of parent-child control.

Allison is totally frustrated and angry with her parents. She's determined to help her father die with dignity and with the most support possible. Yet, whenever she calls (daily) or visits (weekly), her father argues that he's in stable condition and on the road to recovery.

Meanwhile, Allison's mother continues to complain that her father is his own worst enemy, rejecting all the positive things she's doing to help him. Emma often tells Allison that her father actually deserves to suffer because he's so long ignored all the good advice that she, their doctor, and even their friends have given him.

From Allison's perspective, her father is ignoring reality and not planning for his own death. Her mother is hurting as a result of her husband's inevitable impending death and her own anger. And no one is doing any planning that will reduce the amount of pain and uncertainty that's about to happen in their family.

Allison doesn't have power of attorney for either parent, although she's talked about it with both of them a number of times over the past few years. Nor does she have any other legally binding rights to make decisions on behalf of either parent. In short, legally, Allison has no say in what happens with either parent, and that probably won't change.

She's also spoken several times to her parents' family doctor. In his seventies, the doctor treats her the same way her parents do — with a level of disdain and distance, talking down to her rather than with her.

He always concludes conversations with assurances that everything is under control and that he knows what's best for her parents. Meanwhile, in conversations with the case manager at the CCAC, Allison gets the distinct impression that she's talking to a stressed, overworked, well-intentioned but overwhelmed professional who is trying to provide whatever services she can while meeting her many other obligations within the constraints she must face every day.

The Health Care Professional's Point of View

The challenge to children of aging parents is to try to provide care and concern while respecting their parents' wishes to do it their way. When you think about it, it is the same challenge parents face when their children are growing up: to allow them to make decisions and do things that may seem to fly in the face of their best interests and may not reflect the opinions and advice of their parents.

In some child-parent relationships, the conflict in values and opinions is so great that the relationship is disrupted for many years, if not for life. Usually, as children mature, they begin to understand and accept their parents better, and usually, but not always, parents understand their children. Some parents can never get out of the mould of treating their children as children, rather than as adults who happen to be their offspring.

So what can Allison do? First she must accept that the most she can achieve is to give her best care and advice to her parents and then let them make their own decisions, even if she thinks they are not the best ones possible.

In terms of getting that message across to her parents, it would probably be worthwhile to try to meet with them to tell them that, as part of her love and devotion to them, she wants to do whatever she can to help. She can say that her perspective on what is going on may be different from theirs, but that she is willing to accept their views. She should say that while she wants to help, she will not interfere with their decision-making but will be available if necessary when they need her.

Allison might suggest to her mother that blaming her father for what has happened does nothing to help the situation but may in fact make things worse. However, if it is her mother's nature to need to assign blame, then Allison is not going to get very far with that approach. Nevertheless, she must try to focus her mother's efforts on doing what is necessary to make her father as comfortable as possible.

As for the physician, Allison is unlikely to get very far with her pursuits with him. But it may be worthwhile writing to him and thanking him for all the years of support that he has provided to her family. She should express her concerns about her father's present and future needs and at the same time acknowledge that the doctor may understand her father well and that she will trust that he will make the right decisions if and when they are necessary.

Allison also may want to ask the CCAC what kind of home care might be available should her father decide that he does not want to enter a palliative care unit — or for that matter, any other kind of facility — no matter how bad things are.

It is not uncommon for people suffering from cancer to deny the reality of their disease, and trying to convince them of the truth may be counterproductive. Most terminal cancers progress to a point where the symptoms force the person suffering to face the illness.

But the element of hope should never be taken away from someone who realizes that he or she has a terrible disease. For the family that may mean the focus is on relieving symptoms, rather than on trying to cure the disease. Sometimes something urgent or acute happens that shakes the person suffering from the disease into reality. For example, with lung cancer it could be bleeding from the lung. Or it could be evidence that the cancer has spread to the bone, causing great pain, or to the brain, causing seizures or headaches. Whatever it is, the shift in symptoms that cannot be ignored may help everyone focus on the reality of the illness and on the future.

At this point, Allison has to find ways to avoid getting angry with her mother for being angry and frustrated herself. She can be supportive of her mother while not taking on the responsibility of trying to ensure a particular plan of approach. By removing the sense of responsibility for the outcome, Allison may be able to participate in the care of both her father and her mother without feeling that she has failed just because things do not go the way she would want them to go.

Unless there is a sudden turn for the worse, a time will likely come when Allison will be able to provide support and care for her parents. It may be necessary to take a more passive approach right now so that her parents can work out their issues as a couple, however abnormally she may think they are doing it. She should continue to visit on a regular basis but avoid being judgmental when she does. She should call on a periodic basis and, again, listen a lot but not give advice unless it is asked for.

When her parents are ready for her help, she can then be there without resentment. It is crucial for her not to blame them for what has happened and for not allowing her to be involved when she thinks it is necessary. The timing, within reason, has to be their timing, and she has to accept that she can only do what she can do and, of course, what she wants to do, which is to provide the best love and support she can in this very difficult situation.

Meanwhile, Allison should prepare herself for her father's death. One of the difficult tasks that children are likely to face when a parent is nearing the end of life is dealing with the reality and the anticipation of loss while trying to maintain the relationship with the still-living person. Some children and other family members and sometimes friends withdraw from the person as a way of dealing with the coming loss of a loved one. One often hears people who say, "I couldn't face the experience. I would have nothing to say and I was afraid of breaking down." Some individuals find ways to relate and communicate in the deepest and most profound and loving way to their family and friends when they are dying, while others project anger and sorrow and repel those who try to express their love.

Children and other family members must recognize that the knowledge of impending death is not easy, even for the most exceptionally balanced and emotionally secure individuals. It is important to overcome whatever hesitation may exist in visiting and being with the person as he or she nears the end. This time is not about the feelings of the person doing the visiting, but about that of the person who is being visited.

Most people do not want to be alone when they are dying, even though some act in a way that appears to push away even those they love. It is usually valuable to make a point of visiting, and if possible to do so in a predictable fashion so that the person can count on the visit and have something to look forward to. It is not necessary to do anything elaborate when visiting, but sometimes a small gift, especially something the visitor knows the one they are visiting might value, is very much appreciated.

But what does one do during the visit? Just be there. Talk about anything, big or small, but usually personal and on a positive note — what is happening to friends and children that the visitor believes their loved one would enjoy hearing. Bring pictures that reflect good experiences with the intention of helping the person continue to participate in the positive aspects of life. When asked by family members if they should be emotional, I usually tell them if that is the way they feel, then it is okay, but always to remember that it is the person who is ill who is the centre of the exercise, not them. I usually encourage families to let their loved one know just how wonderful a person they are and how meaningful they are and always will be to those who love them.

Lastly, I recommend to families to do as much touching as possible: hold a hand, give a kiss, and provide a soothing massage if that seems to be welcome and helpful. Do not expect the person to respond in kind, which is not important. This is a time for giving on the part of family and friends and not expecting anything in return from the person who is ill and coming to terms with his or her own impending death. After it is over, those who were able to give of themselves and be patient with impatience and express affection and devotion will reap the benefits for many years after the event. They can usually find comfort in the way they behaved at the end, even when the loss is great and the loved one is no longer with them.

Moving On

Living Life without a Loved One

It's not easy learning how to cope with the grieving, how to live on when a spouse or a parent dies, and how to deal with the trauma, guilt, and pain that's involved.

THE CHALLENGE

Marilyn O'Connor is a recent widow. Her husband, Conrad, died six months ago. Although everyone knew that Conrad's death was inevitable and that it was just a matter of how long he could hold out against the pancreatic cancer, his actual passing still came as a shock.

Marilyn, her son, Wes, stepdaughter, Wendy, and their families and several dozen friends attended a graveside service for Conrad on a dreary, overcast fall day with on-again, off-again rain showers that matched their own feelings.

For two months before his death, Conrad had been a patient at a palliative care unit at their local hospital. Marilyn, sixty-eight years old, spent hours with her seventy-two-year-old husband every day. And while many nights she had a series of friends spend time visiting with her and offering support, Marilyn was deeply troubled and very afraid of life without Conrad.

For both, this was their second marriage. Marilyn had left her first husband some three decades ago because of his alcohol problem and her concerns about herself and her son's well-being. She managed to get herself back into the stream of things as a single mother and did well with her new job in an advertising agency.

Conrad's wife died when her car hit black ice on December 24, 1968. She was killed instantly in the crash, but their two-year-old daughter, Wendy, survived with just a few bruises and a long-lasting confusion about what happened to her mother.

Marilyn and Conrad met at a wedding in 1972; she was a friend of the bride and he was a relative of the groom who was at the last moment pressed into serving as best man. It seems the groom and his intended best man had a major disagreement just days before the wedding, and so Conrad was recruited.

A few weeks after meeting at the wedding, Conrad called Marilyn to see if she and her young son would like to join Wendy and him at an Easter egg hunt. So the relationship began, growing into a warm, comfortable friendship, and then into a strong emotional attachment. Two years after meeting — and over time finding that their children got along amazingly well — Conrad proposed. Three months later, they were married at a simple ceremony attended by a handful of friends.

In the years since the marriage, Marilyn and Conrad grew very close to each other and their children. During the summer months, the family often went camping together, and each winter Marilyn and Conrad would go on what they used to call a "just us" holiday for at least a week to a Caribbean island or some other warm vacation spot.

They were not rich, but they were comfortable. Conrad was a partner in a small law firm, and Marilyn continued to work part-time in the creative department of the same advertising agency where she had started after leaving her first husband. Meanwhile, Wes and Wendy emerged as good kids who grew into serious college students and responsible adults. Conrad often told his friends that he and Marilyn were extremely fortunate to have two such wonderful kids.

Wes was married at age thirty to Amy, the daughter of Vietnamese refugees; they have two daughters and live in Edmonton. Wendy was married when she was twenty-seven to Mark, who was just establishing his dentistry practice in Toronto, and four years later she gave birth to their only child, Damian.

Conrad retired precisely on his sixty-fifth birthday; Marilyn had stopped working ten years earlier, instead spending time in volunteer work. Until Conrad was diagnosed with cancer, they travelled as much as possible, played golf together, spent a lot of time hiking in forests, and had a quiet but satisfying social life.

When they retired, Conrad and Marilyn decided to live in Orillia, an hour's drive north of Toronto but within short driving distance of many golf courses and large parks for hiking. The retirement years were good to them, and for them. Conrad, always an animal lover, became involved in the local humane society as a volunteer and fundraiser, but because they wanted to be free to travel they decided not to have an animal of their own.

The pancreatic cancer was a real blow to them all. It was totally unexpected, and right from the outset their family doctor and the oncologist who was seeing Conrad made it clear that the prognosis was very poor. In fact, the oncologist strongly recommended not operating and suggested that any form of treatment was not going to be beneficial in any way. For the first few months, Conrad and Marilyn decided not to tell Wes or Wendy about the cancer, but then thought better of it and explained to them and their spouses, Amy and Mark, exactly what the situation was.

The family rallied in support of Conrad. Amy's and Mark's own parents — with whom they'd always been on very good terms — would call often to see how Conrad was doing, and they stayed in touch with regular emails. Wendy, who lived in Toronto, visited her father every other day and helped her stepmother with housework, and Wes called him at least two or three times a week just for a few minutes.

However, it was clear that Conrad was in a rapid state of decline, with ever-increasing pain that was being treated with increasingly stronger doses of morphine and other pain relievers, given by mouth, injection, or patches. It was also clear that caring for him at home was becoming more and more difficult for Marilyn.

Watching Conrad in his pain and seeing him shrink before their eyes was painful for Marilyn and Wendy. The oncologist finally suggested that they consider placing him in the palliative care unit. This was devastating for Marilyn to hear, but after talking it over with Wendy and Wes, she agreed that it seemed like the best thing to do. Although the admission process was painful to them, the assistance of the unit's social worker, Cynthia, did make some of the decision-making easier.

Near the end, Marilyn was allowed to stay over in the special family room at the palliative care unit. Emotionally she was exhausted, and by the time Conrad died she hardly had any tears left to shed. Cynthia was very supportive of Marilyn, and a few times during the final days she gave Marilyn the opportunity to talk out her feelings about the loss she knew she was going to experience. Wendy had resigned herself to the inevitable but still wanted to find some element of hope to cling to.

Wes flew to Toronto the day his stepfather died, arriving at the palliative care unit just hours before the end. Neither Wendy nor Wes had much contact with Cynthia, although she did offer to meet with them if they wanted to. They declined.

After the funeral, Marilyn found there was a huge empty space in her life. She became withdrawn and very quiet. She rejected her friends' offers of company, choosing instead to spend hours looking at old photos and videos of her holidays with Conrad.

Wendy spent weeks in a very depressed state and kept questioning why her father's condition hadn't been diagnosed sooner and why more couldn't have been done for him. She called her stepmother every day, emailed back and forth with Wes, and found that she was having a difficult time concentrating on her work. Mark offered as much support as possible, but his practice kept him busy six days a week, so he was limited to doing the best he could consoling her and trying to spend more time with Damian.

Three months after the funeral Mark found his wife was still incapable of getting back to what he thought should be their normal life, and he saw that Marilyn was also still in a deep state of grieving. Mark suggested to Wendy that some counselling would be helpful. This caused a huge outburst of anger from Wendy, who lashed out at Mark for not understanding — his parents were still well and together, while her father had died just when he was beginning to enjoy his life.

Wes, meanwhile, seemed more collected, but in their weekly telephone conversations, Mark felt that he, too, was still in pain but just burying it.

THE HEALTH CARE PROFESSIONAL'S POINT OF VIEW

Dealing with death is not easy. It doesn't matter what a person's background and experience might have been, the death of a loved one is a major challenge to a person's equilibrium. However, since death is intrinsic to life, everyone eventually has to come to terms with the realities of someone they love dying.

What can family and friends do to help with the process of bereavement and grief? This is not an easy question to answer, but there are people with a lot of experience in the field and processes that have been proven to be helpful to those going through the experience.

Many religions and cultures have traditions that allow families to mark the various periods of time related to death so that social networks can be re-established with the view of reintegrating family members back into life. In other cultures, the role of the bereaved spouse is almost institutionalized so that there are barriers to reintegration back into the social fabric of the community.

Before anything can be done for Marilyn and her family, someone has to recognize that something is not right and probe possible avenues to improve the situation. The idea is not to try to forget the pain of death and loss, but rather to turn it into something positive that provides a reason once again to participate in life's activities. Many palliative care units, because of their recognition of the difficult path that family members often take after the loss of a loved one, offer bereavement services and counselling to assist family members.

It would have been nice if the palliative care unit where Conrad was a patient had such a program. It may be that it does, but for some reason no contact has been made by the appropriate person to Marilyn or Wendy, as the two of them seem to be having the worse part of the grieving experience. If Wes is the person most likely to be able to take some initiative in helping Marilyn and Wendy to accept assistance, it might be worth his speaking to a member of the palliative care unit's staff to explore what options exist.

Most palliative care programs have social workers involved in the care and support of family members. It is this person, especially if the family has had a good relationship with that person during the dying process, who can become a link in the process of working through the grieving period. Since there was a social worker involved in Conrad's hospitalization, and because Marilyn had the most contact with her, the logical place to start might be to approach Cynthia about the possibility of calling Marilyn. She could ask how things are going and invite Marilyn for a chat as part of the hospital's bereavement program. Wes could call Cynthia and explain what is going on and ask what might be done to help especially Marilyn and Wendy.

Cynthia's overtures might be rebuffed and thought to be intrusive, but most social workers and counsellors who deal with bereavement are pretty good at managing initial rejection of offers of assistance. On the other hand, most people experiencing grief understand that life has to go on and usually respond to gentle and caring overtures of help. Counselling can help to normalize the psychological and physical symptoms often associated with grieving and create a safe environment in which to explore painful feelings. Even when death is expected and family members are prepared for the final event, the grief reaction may not be any less intense or prolonged than when a death is sudden.

Loving and caring family members can be instrumental in such assistance, although the kind of response that Mark experienced from Wendy is not unusual. The timing of the next attempt to discuss the issue has to be carefully considered and prepared for and could be couched in the desire to help deal with the next stages of life. Mark has to be sensitive to Wendy's sensibilities, but he can build on being able to help her stepmother, while being available for each other and their child.

Each situation is different, but the goal has to be to regain meaning in life, which does not imply forgetting the person who has died and who was loved. Sometimes a way can be found to commemorate the person who died that will give extra meaning to survivors. That is often why endowment funds for students, projects, or donations to charitable societies are suggested as a way of remembering the life of a loved one.

The wife of one of my patients decided to set up an endowment fund in her husband's name for the psychiatry unit that was so helpful in his overcoming severe depression. He spoke about it very highly after he recovered from his mental illness, prior to his death from another cause. In addition, she decided to become a volunteer at the hospital in which the psychiatry unit was located so that she could help other people.

In this case, Marilyn might want to consider setting up a fund for the palliative care unit to provide a better place for families to stay during the final days of their loved one's life. Or she might offer to work for the Cancer Society as a canvasser or in its office. This kind of work often allows for relationships to develop with other people who have lost loved ones to cancer; this common bond against the enemy of cancer often leads to social involvement.

Another option might be for Marilyn to get involved with the humane society as Conrad had, and continue with an activity that was dear to his heart. Similar options might be attractive to Wendy, although the main focus appears to be to meet Marilyn's needs. It is possible that if her needs are met, Wendy will refocus her energies on the future rather than on the past.

Whatever is done, the family has to be sensitive to the needs of Marilyn and Wendy, especially as they seem to be having the greatest difficulty. It is not that Wes would not benefit from bereavement counselling, it is just that he may have to get involved after the pattern and process is already established with his mother and sister.

The goal, of course, is to get on with life, because that is what life is all about. Those people who do not accomplish that goal often become embittered and lose the ability to enjoy and share life with others.

If Conrad knew what was happening, it seems likely that he would tell his family to remember him as someone who enjoyed life and that he would want them to continue to live in a loving and expansive way. His death should be a catalyst to them to remember the wonderful things in life and to strive to enjoy them rather than a reason to dwell on the past and the sadness that it contains.

Roz and Max

by Michael Gordon

My father's voice was shaky. "Mommy had a little stroke and is in the hospital. They called it a 'transient' attack." My eighty-two-year-old father, Max, was calling me in Toronto from Brooklyn, where he and my mother, Roslyn (Roz), also eighty-two, lived together in the cottage-like home they had owned for almost forty years. He explained that my mother had suddenly had trouble speaking and her face had gone crooked. By the time she arrived at the hospital by ambulance she had recovered, but she was admitted for testing.

As a geriatrician practising in Toronto I knew that my mother, a diabetic, had atrial fibrillation and was at risk for a so-called embolic stroke (blood clot to the brain). The cardiologist explained that her CT scan was normal and that he had anticoagulated (thinned) her blood. He was trying to convince her to go on a long-acting anticoagulant, called Warfarin, but she was adamant that she didn't want that drug because of the risks of bleeding and the need for frequent blood tests.

I was not surprised that my mother, a very active and spry person, would not want to be encumbered by frequent tests and doctors' visits.

When I called her, she said she was fine and wanted to go home. "The food is lousy and they keep sending me for tests," she complained. The cardiologist recommended putting her on Aspirin, which is also used to decrease the risk of blood clots. It isn't the ideal drug treatment, but, at the time, the more recent studies showing the benefits of Warfarin were not yet in the mainstream medical literature. I reluctantly agreed to his decision and felt that I should not influence my mother against her wishes to take a treatment that had substantial side effects.

Immediately upon exiting the hospital parking lot, my mother, eager to leap back into the stream of her activities, insisted on dropping in to visit an ailing relative. "Can you imagine," she recounted to me, "that I caught my foot in the car door and fell and banged my knee! I look like a school kid — all black and blue." What relief I felt that she was not on Warfarin; she would have bled profusely from the fall. It seemed so incongruent that my mother, such a graceful and fluid dancer, had a propensity to fall! This tendency, and her level of activity at her local seniors' centre, meant that anticoagulant therapy would be highly risky for her. Her cardiologist's decision appeared to be the right one.

During the next few weeks, each time I spoke to my mother, who said she was fine and active and dancing away at the seniors' centre, I felt relieved at the decision that had been made. Then came the distraught call from my father: "Mommy collapsed and I called 911. I couldn't move her from the bathroom — she is in the hospital." She was at a local city hospital, not the HMO (Health Maintenance Organization) hospital where she previously had been a patient.

I called my sister, Diti (a nickname for Diane), in Chicago and we coordinated our flights to New York. The taxi ride from LaGuardia to the house in Brighton Beach was filled with scenes remembered from childhood as we passed familiar landmarks. We got closer to our house and I recognized the bicycle path where my father took Diti and me for long bike rides when we were youngsters.

The news at the emergency department was shattering. My mother had had a massive left CVA (stroke), leaving her paralyzed down the right side of her body and requiring ventilator-assisted breathing. It was the beginning of the Memorial Day weekend in May, with the hospital short-staffed and frenzied and the emergency room a holding pen until beds on wards became available. And there lay my mother amidst beds and stretchers of bodies, on a ventilator, suddenly so frail and helpless. I took my father's hand as we approached her bedside. It was impossible to reconcile this scene with the images of my gregarious mother, twirling across the dance floor with vibrancy and joy. I gazed at her, and in that instant I realized that our lives with my mother would never again be the same. I clung to echoes of her laughter as she would tell a story or watch the antics of my children. I knew that my beloved mother had a tough and uncertain road ahead.

At home my father explained the events again: "She was in the bathroom, all dressed up getting ready to go to the centre, when I heard a scream and a bang, like something falling. I had trouble pulling her out of the bathroom and used the bathroom rug under her to help move her. I dragged her out of the bathroom but I couldn't get her up. I called 911 and they rushed her to the hospital.

"She hadn't been feeling that well but insisted on going to the centre. I told her she shouldn't go because she might collapse on the way — and then it happened in the house."

In a way it was comforting to know that, up to the very moment she was felled by the stroke, my mother was enjoying her active life.

My mother was moved to a six-bed hospital room, and the nurse reported that she had opened her eyes for a moment a bit earlier but had not responded to her name. The CT scan confirmed the stroke, and a program to anticoagulate her blood was started. I was a bit shocked that she was on a ventilator on a regular medical floor, rather than in the intensive care unit (ICU). But the medical resident explained that there were no ICU beds and they thought it was best to move her out of the emergency room. We arranged for private duty nursing to supplement the regular nursing staff, which we could see was inadequate for the task at hand.

I noticed that my mother was on a regular mattress and asked about moving her to a pressure-reducing one. The nurse said, "This is the Memorial Day weekend, and we can't get a pressure-reducing mattress until Tuesday." I was really worried about her developing a pressure ulcer from being immobilized for three days, but the nurse reiterated that there was nothing she could do. She promised that the nurses would shift her position as frequently as they could. The problem seemed to reflect the condition of the whole hospital, which was rundown, having been built sometime when I was a youngster in the 1950s. Now, like many of New York's city hospitals, it was understaffed and dilapidated.

We all sat around the bed and took turns going out, walking around the hospital floor and going down to the coffee shop, not knowing if Roz was going to survive and, if so, what kind of recovery she would make. On Sunday morning my mother opened her eyes and, with apparent recognition, tried to talk but could not because of the tube in her throat. Her right side was completely paralyzed and her face was drooping, but at least her eyes were open and she seemed to be able to focus on us and follow our conversation. She indicated that the tube was bothering her. The doctor said he was going to try to remove it and hoped that she could breathe on her own. When the tube came out it was wonderful to see her whole face. She tried to speak, but couldn't because of the stroke. My father left the room and started crying in the corridor. Diti and I held him and told him that we would do whatever it would take to get her better.

The next few months were full of both hope and despair, with endless physical and emotional stress, as Diti and I alternated or overlapped our visits to Brooklyn. Supporting my father on the phone was not easy; he was despondent. With every small improvement he was hopeful, and with every small setback he was devastated. There were moments of humour and pathos, deep drama, and the sharing of basic human emotion with other families whose loved ones shared the various hospital rooms with my mother. One time, soon after the ventilator was removed, my mother indicated by scrawling with her left hand that she wanted a cup of coffee, or as she would have said in her Brooklynese, a "cuppa cawfee." My mother loved coffee, and it was a joy to provide her with a cup, even if it went through the feeding tube. It was only after that tube was finally removed that she was able to drink some coffee very slowly through a straw and enjoy its taste.

My mother played the piano and was an accomplished ballet dancer in her youth and as an adult. She was a devotee of dance and music. As children, even though we did not have a lot of money, my mother made sure Diti and I had music lessons and often took us to concerts, shows, and ballet performances, which we enjoyed even though we always had the least expensive seats. Those times were special experiences in my life and set the stage for my own lifelong appreciation of music and dance.

I thought that bringing music to her would be therapeutic. We bought a portable tape recorder with earphones and put on Tschaikowsky's Nutcracker Suite. Her face lit up and she started moving her good hand and her head rhythmically to the music. Most poignant was that she started pointing the toe of her left foot the way a dancer does. We went through tape after tape, my mother responding to music that I knew she loved: Gershwin, Mozart, Beethoven, and one of my favourites, Rachmaninov, whose second piano concerto was one of the first records our family ever owned. She kept the earphones on through-out most of the day, and we instructed the privately hired caregivers to keep the music going. It added meaning to my mother's day, and with-out it she had little to look forward to.

She had some major setbacks: a week after she was admitted a blood clot lodged in her left leg, and Diti struggled to get urgent medical help.

Emergency surgery successfully removed the clot and appeared to salvage the leg. It was during that time of post-operative intensive care admission that the most terrible outcome of her hospitalization fully developed: a terrible deep and painful pressure ulcer on the lower part of her backside. During this period, we became very close as a family, dealing with fears and hopes and sleeping again in the very small home that we grew up in. Diti and I strengthened an already great and affec-tionate respect for each other. It was an unfortunately painful way of enriching our close and loving relationship.

We optimistically welcomed my mother's transfer to the hospital's rehabilitation unit. We began to fantasize that she would go home, and we began to explore what it would take to modify the little house to accommodate her. How would my father, who had significant angina, be able to care for her? We explored how much outside help would be required in the home but also looked at nursing homes in Brooklyn. Diti investigated nursing homes in her neighbourhood of Oak Park, Illinois, thinking that both my parents could move there. We even looked into how she could be moved by an air ambulance. At one point my father almost accusingly asked me why I could not get her into the geriatric centre where I worked in Canada. I explained the immigration issues, but because he persisted I looked into it and was told that we could not take an ill person into the country, even with monetary guarantees, because of the high financial risk to the publicly funded health care system. It was when I was in the process of exploring this option further that my mother's condition suddenly got worse with the development of gangrene in her left, non-paralyzed leg.

When the gangrene was diagnosed the surgeon told us she would need a leg amputation at least above the knee, if not at the hip, depending on what transpired. This would mean she would be left with a completely paralyzed right leg and little or no left leg. It was hard for us to imagine that Roz, a person who loved to dance and move to music, would have agreed to such a state of affairs if she had been able to discuss it with us. Since she'd had her stroke, we could not really communicate effectively with her, but we did the best we could as a loving family who felt we understood her values.

We had arranged for Jessica, a wonderful woman who had looked after another family member for years, to assist in her care and feeding, as our HMO would no longer approve private duty nursing. We observed that the unit nurses were too busy to provide adequate care. The knowledge that a loving and caring person was with her for many hours during the evening and night, especially when Diti and I were not in New York, was very comforting.

Then came the ultimate choice. My mother required morphine to quell the pain from her gangrenous leg and from the deep pressure ulcer. Her level of consciousness varied, but through moaning and grimacing when she was awake she indicated that she had terrible pain. Diti, my father, and I struggled with the decision. It was impossible to imagine her living with the expected state of leg paralysis and the amputation. With heart-wrenching effort we decided to decline surgery but rather to treat her with painkillers and let nature take its course.

The physician suggested putting in a feeding tube, but we decided that it would prolong her agony and we rejected that as well. The doctor, who had palliative care experience, sympathetically agreed with us, but some of the nurses accepted the decision only reluctantly. One nursing supervisor had the audacity and insensitivity to ask me why I was "starving my mother to death" by not putting in a feeding tube. I had to control my rage when I explained that our family wanted my mother to have as peaceful a death as possible under the circumstances.

I spoke to the doctor, who concurred with our request to treat my mother palliatively, using morphine round the clock as is done with patients dying from cancer. Despite the medical order, it soon became apparent that the nurses kept waiting for my mother to express pain before giving her the injection. Diti or I had to persistently ask, sometimes almost beg, the nurses to give her the morphine at the appointed time and reiterate that the order read "every four hours round the clock," not "as required," the latter being the usual non-palliative morphine order.

The vigil began. My father had the greatest difficulty watching her suffer, and we generally did not leave him alone in her room. Diti or I sat with our mother for hours on end, listening to her rhythmic breathing, with the rasping sound from secretions gathering in her chest. She was not awake and did not seem to hear what we said even though we spoke to her of our love for her. I put the earphones from the tape recorder on my head and turned on Rachmaninov's second piano concerto. That piece has had a profound affect on me since the first time I heard it in our one-bedroom apartment in Brighton Beach when I was about seven years old. It sustained me through medical school, and now I listened to it over and over again as it wove itself into my mother's laboured breathing.

Exhausted, we decided to go home for the night. Jessica was to stay there to be with Roz. Early in the morning, Jessica called with the news: "Come to the hospital now; it's over." Sadly my mother died with Jessica, rather than with any of her family, by her side. Diti and I went to the hospital. Our mother was lying in the bed, uncovered, with an ECG machine connected to her, a last rites ritual of a medical system that seemed to forget dignity but was enthralled with technology. I started pulling out the intravenous line, and the nurse began to object. I firmly told her I was a physician and her son and could not bear seeing her in this undignified condition, uncovered and with tubes connected to her. Neither the on-call physician nor any of the nurses uttered a word of condolence. It was just business as usual. We covered her with the sheet and collected the few items from her side table and went to the office to sign the papers. Her ordeal was over. The ten weeks of coming and going as the long-distance son and daughter was over. Now there was only my father, in the small bungalow that had been our home and now was his alone.

After the funeral and the mourning period, we tried to help my father organize and clean the house. He said he wanted to stay there and assured us that he would be fine. One of us called almost every day.

The few friends and neighbours and his sister who lived in Queens tried to lend a hand, but mostly he wanted to be left alone. We knew he was shopping for groceries because the supermarket debits showed up on the credit card, which he shared with Diti. He rejected the idea of rejoining the seniors' centre and claimed he had gone there only to please Roz. We figured the real reason he refused to go was that he was afraid that he would break down and start crying, something he did whenever he talked about our mother.

Our periodic visits revealed that he was managing, but the state of the house was deteriorating. He rejected any outside help in cleaning or cooking. We thought he might be depressed, but with time he seemed to express his normal interest in reading his papers, especially the financial sections, and he watched television. He continued to visit some friends from the seniors' centre but refused to attend any activities despite urging from everyone. He rejected most invitations to join his sister in a meal, but when Diti or I visited he would agree to eat out with us and his sister and her husband and seemed to enjoy himself.

We struggled with his future, even though he said he was fine. I decided to try to get him resident status in Canada. My father agreed to apply, acknowledging how much he and Roz enjoyed their frequent visits to Toronto. After the certificate allowing him entry arrived, he said, "I'm not sure I am going to move. Will I have to take a new driving test?" I could not answer for sure but was pretty certain that he would eventually have to qualify for an Ontario licence. He expressed reluctance to submit to reapplying for a licence, as he was concerned that he might fail the test.

During a visit to Toronto he expressed other doubts. "You know I will probably have to pay more income tax in Canada," he commented.

"But you get more in the way of services here," I replied.

"What kind of services do I need?" he asked.

I reminded him of the cost of the long-term care facility that we visited when Roz was sick, and he nodded in agreement. But after the week-long visit, he was eager to go home, and once there he said he wasn't ready to move. I tried to cajole him, reminding him how hard it was to look after Roz with us being so far away.

"I understand, but I can't make the move yet," he replied. His certificate of immigration expired. He was staying at the bungalow in Brooklyn. Diti and I reluctantly agreed that he had to do it his way.

He occasionally visited me in Toronto or Diti in Chicago. During each visit he seemed a little more frail, but he was still independent in all of his activities. He became increasingly sloppy, but that had always been part of his character. We enjoyed his visits, and he took pride in seeing his grandchildren and experiencing some of their activities like hockey games and their playing their musical instruments. But he was always eager to return; sometimes he suggested he would cut his usual week-long visit short, agreeing to stay the full week only when I told him the cost of changing his flight.

The house in Brooklyn was looking worse and worse. He tried to fix the bathroom shower faucets but succeeded in breaking the wall in the process. The float in the toilet broke, and being the engineer, do-it-yourself expert, he fixed it by rigging a primitive combination of clips that could be pulled in order to flush. He became embroiled in a lawsuit with a neighbour whose new medical building compromised his ability to use the house's side entrance. That five-year legal case became the focus of all of his psychological energies, and most telephone conversations centred around the topic. The case was finally settled out of court, although my father was never satisfied and complained he never had his "day in court." We visited to celebrate his eighty-ninth birthday. Diti arranged a dinner with his sister and her husband. On the way to the restaurant we stopped to buy him a new television as a birthday gift. At dinner, he ate well, but slowly and very tentatively. Afterwards, when he was alone with Diti as the rest of us went to get the car, he turned to her and asked, "How did I get here?" Diti and I took him home and noticed some over-the-counter sleeping medications on his bedside table. Because of a recent episode of low back pain, his physician had given him some strong analgesics.

During this visit, Diti and I noted the dramatic deterioration in my father's functioning. The house was a complete disaster. There were mouse droppings everywhere. We found multiple cheques written for the same bill, each addressed but not sent out. And we found monthly cheques made out to a charity, but not one that had ever been special to him. It seemed he had forgotten to whom he had sent money. He admitted to falling a couple of times and had recently hit his head and cut his forehead. He blamed it on tripping because of the clutter in the house.

Diti and I agreed that the decision could no longer be left to him. Diti said, "We are moving you to Chicago." We waited for his standard adamant refusal. Instead, he nodded in agreement. Diti told him she would go back to Chicago and see what was available that would provide independence and privacy. He agreed again.

It was now Diti's turn to go through the process of thinking about how and where to move my father. With great luck she found availability in a retirement home five minutes from where she lived. Three weeks later, we both returned to Brooklyn to help him move. The plan was for Diti to drive to Chicago with our father in his small car. We spent a weekend trying to clean up the house but mainly identifying the papers and personal effects that he would want to take with him. We lined the streets with green garbage bags filled with things we had decided could be tossed.

It wasn't easy to identify essential papers, income tax forms that had not been filed, and bills that hadn't been paid. But gradually things fell into place, and Diti and my father were ready to leave. At first, he climbed into the driver's seat, saying he would drive because he knew the route better than Diti. I was concerned that he would actually insist on driving, but Diti managed the scene by gently saying, "You can't drive, I need you to navigate." And with that she held his hand to help him out of the driver's side of the car, put him in the other side, and gave him the maps. He seemed satisfied in this role.

That night I received a call from Diti. "What a trip," my sister laughingly said. "First of all it took two hours to get out of New York because although Daddy thinks he can navigate and I assumed he could, we got lost a few times before we got on the highway." She continued, "Then the fun began. It was like travelling with a two-year-old just recently potty trained. I drove into every rest stop and insisted that he go to the bathroom. It made for a very long trip. His back was hurting and he really was slow, so I had to pull him out of the car, hold his hand to go to the bathroom, and help him back. He kept asking if I was tired, offering to drive." I was relieved that they had made it to the halfway mark only a little later than expected. Diti went on, "Daddy thinks this is a pretty swanky motel because it's a cut above the Motel 6 he's used to, although it's not really that fancy. But he thinks it's great. He even asked if it has a casino and said if I want some money to gamble he would give it to me." We both roared with laughter.

The next night I spoke to Diti again. "We made it, but it was a trip that was so exhausting I cannot believe I did it." I asked if he recognized the neighbourhood when they drove through it even though he had not been there for some years. "Oh yes. He named the streets and started giving me directions on how to get to the house. He asked about the shops and was surprised when I told him that some of them were no longer in business."

His apartment at the retirement community had been newly painted and carpeted. It was nicely furnished and even had paintings on the walls, and it had a lovely modern kitchen. Diti and I assured him that we would not sell the house unless he wanted to, but reminded him that he had to make a minimum five-month commitment to the apartment. Diti asked the home to furnish an extra bed so that she could stay over on a moment's notice, if necessary, which my father liked.

After two weeks, in keeping with my father's independent, stubborn nature, he declared he was ready to go back home to Brooklyn. Diti reminded him that he had agreed to stay five months and that he would be obligated to pay for the apartment whether or not he stayed.

Diti visited him several times a day during those first weeks to help him acclimatize, often staying with him during the daily luncheon program on his floor. She sat with him and engaged others in conversation to break the ice and help him meet people. She placed his medications in a pillbox to prevent the kinds of mix-ups we suspected had been happening in Brooklyn. When she couldn't visit, she called to do everything to encourage the success of his move.

The township offered a program of discounted meals at local restaurants for seniors. Max loved this program and especially enjoyed one restaurant that offered good food and ample neighbourhood action. The waitresses began to know him, remembering that he preferred soup, not salad, along with his french fries, chocolate ice cream, and tea. Diti thanked the restaurant owner for helping our father to adjust and see what a wonderful place Oak Park was. Max, a true product of the Depression, appreciated being served a $10 meal for $3. He began to say what a nice neighbourhood he now lived in.

One evening he called Diti saying he was feeling really bad. He was having a terrible bout with constipation — something that had plagued him for many years in Brooklyn — and said he needed to go to the hospital.

Thinking a trip to the hospital wasn't necessary, Diti instead gave him water, stool softeners, and watermelon as he sat on the toilet. He used glycerine suppositories and finally was successful. Diti stayed overnight on the bed set up for just such a situation. The next day, she was able to challenge his thought that maybe he could go back to Brooklyn. She asked him, "What would you have done last night if I hadn't been five minutes away?" He conceded. This was the turning point to his agreeing to the permanency of the move.

Diti knew that he was making a very positive adjustment when he began to relay details of conversations he was having on his own with people in the lunchroom. Sometimes he would read his *New York Times* (he was the only resident getting this paper delivered) in the lounge rather than going back to his apartment. He always wore a baseball cap that had Indiana written on it, and he found that it provided a nice icebreaker, as people would ask him if he was from Indiana. In his most engaging way he'd say, "No, but I passed through it on my way from New York." Diti was able to lessen her visits to once a day and then occasionally missing a day here or there. He would tell people that Diti had "shanghaied" him, and she would retort, "No, I kidnapped him." After three months in the apartment, he announced he wanted to visit Brooklyn. His decision to move had happened so fast that there were people to whom he hadn't said goodbye. He worried they would wonder why he never answered his telephone.

Diti took him home and they visited the few really special friends he had left behind. He repeatedly described his new living arrangement in Oak Park very positively. At the end of the Brooklyn visit he said, "I am ready to sell the house." We were ecstatic! Fortunately, the next-door neighbour was a realtor, and before they returned to Chicago a contract was signed. My father conceded that life in Oak Park was a much easier and nicer life than he had had in Brooklyn during the previous few years.

One month after the move, his new medical insurance was in place. He had a complete medical examination by a colleague of mine and his medications were modified so that many of the problems that plagued him in Brooklyn, like his back pain, were brought under control.

To our delight, with these changes and some additional medications that he needed, his mental state improved remarkably, as did his mood and interactions.

A few more months passed, including the Chicago winter, and my father settled in nicely at the retirement home. He gradually began to participate in the various social activities. Each phone call seemed more positive, and Diti said he admitted that he had been doing very poorly in Brooklyn and expressed gratitude that we had "forced" him to move. He even said, "You saved my life." I found phone conversations to be like years ago. I could discuss world events and politics. One Sunday evening I asked him about what was in the *Times* and he said, "I don't get the *Times* any more." I asked with concern, "Why not, are you having trouble reading it?" (This was a man who had read the *New York Times* every day of his adult life.) "No," he replied, "I started getting the *Chicago Tribune* instead because it has local news. I thought it was worth knowing what's going on here." To me that was the best indicator that he was staying in Chicago and that his mental function was probably as good as anyone could possibly hope for.

The issue of his driving came up from time to time. We had made a decision not to allow him to drive, and Diti kept his car in her driveway. In reality he had no reason to drive, but as is often the case, he considered not driving as a serious blow to his independence. We understood the impact that the loss of his licence might have for him, so we agreed to look into the Chicago regulations, hoping that with time it would become less and less of an issue. His insurance was changed from New York to Illinois, and he saved thousands of dollars with that alone.

We got him new Illinois plates — handicapped ones because of his bad back and angina — but put off applying for a new licence. A couple of times Diti took him for his favourite drive to the country and found a secluded place to let him drive. Each time, after no more than fifteen minutes, he was tired and willing to give up the wheel.

Things were progressing very well, with most of the details of my father's health gradually being addressed. One of the outstanding issues was his hearing. He had been resistant to wearing a hearing aid even though it was clear to everyone around him that he had hearing problems. We modified his phone and encouraged him to seek advice, which he refused. On one of his visits to Toronto I arranged for him to have an excellent hearing evaluation at the Baycrest Centre for Geriatric Care, where I work. The audiologist was very perceptive when she responded to his statement, "My hearing is fine, you know." She showed him the audiogram, appealing to his engineering expertise, and said, "Mr. Gordon, you are correct that your hearing is okay, but you have major problems with discrimination of sound. Although you might hear the sound, you cannot figure out its meaning." He accepted the explanation but later on again declined consideration of a hearing aid, saying that it was not necessary. Meanwhile Diti and I struggled with telephone conversations, repeating ourselves many times and speaking slowly when it was clear that my father had failed to understand what we had told him.

Then, in March 2001, on a Friday just prior to my family's winter ski vacation, I received a call from Diti: "Daddy fell this morning in the bathroom, but he seems okay and I am taking him for his scheduled hearing aid assessment." That appointment turned out to be fortuitous.

While registering at the local hospital for the assessment, Max had a momentary seizure-like episode. His face grimaced, his left arm went up involuntarily, and Diti screamed for help. He was immediately transferred to the hospital's next-door emergency room.

The nurse picked up the phone as my father was being hooked up to the cardiac monitor and said to me, "The tracing looks to me like he is in some kind of heart block." The next day, the cardiologist confirmed that he might need a pacemaker but wanted to observe him further over the weekend to make sure the problem was not related to any of his medications. I assured Diti and my father that should he need a pacemaker the procedure was very safe and effective. By this time my family and I were in Quebec on our holiday. While my wife and children were out skiing, I stayed at the condo and did my writing and reading, staying close to the phone.

The day after the pacemaker was inserted, my father had an episode of vague chest pain, which turned out to be a small heart attack. The medical team at first thought that he could be treated with an angioplasty (a balloon widening of the heart's blood vessels), but it soon became clear that he would require urgent bypass surgery.

I explained the urgency and poor prognosis without surgery to my father over the phone. He said, "Let me think about it." I replied, "You have about five minutes to think because if it's not done you probably won't be around for very long." He said, with hardly a moment's hesitation, "Okay, if that's the case." Surgery was booked for the day we were driving back to Toronto.

There was no way I could get to Chicago to be with him, but I spoke to him the night before and I arranged a flight for the next morning. Diti kept me posted during the drive.

Max had indicated to Diti what outcome he would accept from his surgery and what limits he would want on care should it not be successful. I was very concerned about the possible deleterious effects of major surgery on his mental function, but other than a short period of confusion related to the pain medications, his mind was quite clear. He even started making humorous remarks to the nurses, who appeared to thoroughly enjoy him. They were all very impressed with his rapid mental and physical recovery. Within the week he was on the rehabilitation unit. Two more weeks and he was sent back to his retirement home. He now knew, for sure, that his move to Oak Park had literally saved his life.

With his ninetieth birthday coming up, I planned a visit to help celebrate. It coincided with a conference on aging in Chicago, so I took advantage of the opportunity to work and celebrate at the same time. The three of us went out for dinner, and after the meal my father said, "I want to see if after I eat and walk I get chest pain the way I used to." I remember those years when my father would stop before he went for a walk to "catch his breath" and usually take a nitroglycerine pill to relieve his angina. We walked up the street and then down and my father said, "I don't feel anything; the surgery really worked." Of course he had not had the surgery because of angina but rather because of the small heart attack, but a "side effect" of the surgery was improvement of his angina.

Soon after, an offer came through on the house, and Diti and I were confronted with the prospect of actually cleaning the place. We knew that my parents had saved almost everything, so the task of making it ready for possession was not pleasant and loomed over us. We had planned to bring my father down to see the house again before we emptied it, but because of his heart surgery we had to cancel that plan. It was, therefore, left to Diti and me to do the job. I suggested that we just hire a dumpster and have the house emptied. Diti, rightfully as I soon learned, disagreed.

It was late Friday night when I arrived. Diti had already packed many bags with clothes and an equal number with garbage, gradually emptying overfilled cupboards and dressers, of which my parents had many. At one point she stopped and asked, "So you want to just throw everything out?" as she handed me my original birth certificate, which she had plucked from between some old papers stuffed in one of the dresser drawers. Although I had long ago obtained a copy of it, I held the original in my hand and wondered what other treasures we might find in the little three-bedroom bungalow.

Each item resulted in a comment or observation, and some past association was evoked. There was no rhyme or reason to where things had been stored. A box of childhood and family pictures was in one drawer; Diti's Grade 5 school essay was in another; my high school yearbook was in yet another. We found the bill of sale for the Sohmer baby grand piano that our grandmother purchased for our mother in 1935, the one on which I learned to play. We found the receipts of the mother's milk our parents had to purchase after I was born prematurely because I could not tolerate anything else.

We found a letter from our bubbie (grandmother) to our mother, then pregnant with Diti and still in Dearborn, Michigan. It assured her that we could live with her in her Brighton Beach apartment and that my mother needn't wait until my father's transfer from Dearborn, where he worked for the U.S. Department of Defense. The letter brought back memories of the apartment we lived in before we moved into the house: the large single bedroom where Diti and I and our bubbie slept, our parents sleeping in the living room with a bookcase separating their "bedroom" area from the rest of the living room, which contained the baby grand piano, a sofa, and some chairs.

The most poignant discovery was a typewritten letter from our mother to her father, who had unfortunately abandoned the family to pursue another relationship. The letter pleaded with him to be the father she remembered — when her mother sang opera and he played the English concertina. The letter brought us to tears as we read of the pain she struggled with in trying to come to terms with the problematic relationship she had with her father. It also left us puzzled because our mother had never typed. We wondered who might have helped her write this letter. We couldn't know if it was ever actually sent and we were looking at a copy, or if she had never mailed it to him. It reminded us painfully of the absence of our mother and the many struggles of her life. We could not ask her questions about the letter.

As we found other things, we were grateful that we were doing this job while our father was still alive. Later we could ask him who people were in old photographs or named in documents. I asked about a hospital record we found showing that I had required a blood transfusion as a premature baby. He confirmed that the blood for the transfusion came directly from him to me — the way all transfusions were done in 1941. The scar at the elbow crease of my left arm from that transfusion has often been the subject of conversation whenever I donated blood.

We found a document required by Max for work that listed all the personal details of immediate relatives, including dates of birth and city and country of origin. It was a wonderful record of our family history, confirming our Jewish Lithuanian heritage and showing that our name, Gordon, had never been changed as so many other immigrant names had. As well, this document confirmed the Scottish link to our name, something I had discovered years before while studying in Scotland.

We were very happy to find pictures of our mother in her youth in artistic poses from her ballet and interpretative dancing days. Other pictures much later in her life were of her dancing at the local senior citizens' centre, which was such an important focal point of her life. Although she gave up professional dancing aspirations when she got married, throughout her lifetime she and my father would be the subject of much admiration whenever they danced together in public. I recall at my wedding in Winnipeg to my wife, Gilda, how guests remarked to me how wonderfully they danced and especially how expressively and beautifully my mother moved. At the retirement home, my father still was able to take part in the social dances, and Diti has danced with him when he was ninety.

She recognizes that being able to dance with him is a great gift and part of the legacy from his life with our mother. We slogged along filling bags and showing each other nostalgic finds, always making sure that anything my father might want or need was kept. We called him occasionally to ask if we could throw out some item or other. He asked us to keep some old *New York Times* clippings, as he wanted to read them again.

On the second day of our cleanup, Diti yelled from the basement that she had found something special and chided me again for having suggested that we just call in a hauling company to take everything. It was two huge boxes of personal letters. It seemed like every letter ever exchanged among us was in these boxes. There were hundreds, including those from my six-month trip to Europe when I was nineteen years old and many more from my six years of medical studies in Scotland, my one year as a draft-dodging landed immigrant in Montreal, and my four years living in Israel. There were letters from the two years that Diti spent in the Peace Corps in Tunisia. There were letters from old friends.

We started reading them, some to each other when we shared the person or the experience, and some on our own, because they were very personal.

The letter that caused both Diti and I to laugh most together was one she wrote from summer camp when she was fourteen years old. In it, the essence of her intelligence, sensitivity, and maturity came out loud and clear, and within its commentaries and questions was evidence that our relationship was built on and continues to flourish because of the strong values and trust that our parents had in the two of us. Cleaning the house increased the bonds that tie the two of us and made us realize even more that the legacy of our parents is imprinted indelibly upon us.

Finally, we finished the job, had a few more visits to get the house ready for everything that was headed for the dumpster that was eventually required, and closed the deal. The home of our youth was no longer ours. My father no longer had a place to return to in Brooklyn. Chicago was now his home, and at least he had Diti (whom I had renamed "Deity" in honour of her divine devotion to our father) close to him to help him care for himself. I was still the distant son, trying to be of assistance by phone and the occasional visit and through very close communication with Diti.

She has assumed the major part of caregiving. She has done it all with the greatest love and devotion that anyone could ever expect from a child. We have concluded that it is all part of being a caring and loving family and that there really could and should not be any other way, although we know that many times things do not work out so well in families.

My father has come through a lot. Now we just take it one day at a time and enjoy the fact that he has a life with a lot of interests and satisfactions and that we are still able to enjoy his presence, his humour, and his still sweet and engaging personality.

AN UPDATE: THE PRESENT

Since his heart surgery, my father has done quite well, with the past three years being ones of relative stability and enjoyment. He has accommodated to the retirement home, and the staff has clearly developed a special fondness for him. I knew that he was comfortable in his new home when, on one of my visits, I arrived early enough on a Friday that I had chance to join him for the community member lunch program. This program, sponsored by a grant from the city council, allows people from the community to dine at bargain prices in a dining area rented from the retirement home. The convenience (it is located on the floor my father lives on), bargain prices, and outside company all make this program very attractive to my father.

As we walked into the room filled with tables and diners, with my father wearing his ubiquitous baseball hat, many called over, "Hey Max, sit here. Is that your son?" We eventually picked a table with a few other lunch program participants and I found that they all knew almost everything about me. Clearly my father was a favourite among the diners, but he must have spoken often about me, as they were right up to date with my personal and professional life. I must admit, it was a very warm feeling to know that they knew of me through him, who, unlike my mother who loved to talk about me to anyone, anywhere, had always been a more reserved person when it came to referring to his children. The fact that everyone knew Diti because of her frequent visits clearly was an entrance point to their knowing more about me, the "famous" doctor/son from Toronto.

Another year has passed and I watch my father gradually physically slowing up. Although he can still manage most things and he attends the retirement home's social events often with Diti, his gait is slower and more deliberate. On one of my visits, I told Diti that I wanted to have a talk with him again with her in attendance about his future wishes should he become ill. Even though there was nothing pressing at the moment, I wanted us all to be clear as to what his wishes might be for future care if there were a crisis or terrible affliction. So after lunch we went back to Diti's home. We were sitting on the sofa and easy chair, my ninety-one-year-old father, my sister, and me, and we started to speak.

I reminded him that we had actually talked about his wishes some years ago while walking on the boardwalk in Brighton Beach where he was still living at the time. I was reminding him of our painful experience with the terrible way "Mommy" had died during her final illness and how much I would like to avoid anything like that with him should something just as terrible happen. I asked my father on that quite balmy spring day what he would want in a comparable circumstance. After a few moments of silence, I outlined to him what I thought his values were based on my knowledge of him and through observing him as the suffering husband of our ailing mother. I told him I thought he would not want "heroics" if he could not make a good recovery. He answered, "Exactly." That was how things stood in terms of communication until this Saturday afternoon in Chicago when Diti and I were going to speak to him on the subject again with both of us present.

My sister and I had decided that we should have an open heart-to-heart talk with him so we could be sure about his wishes and desires for the future, even though he had recovered wonderfully from his bypass surgery and was managing very well in his new environment, being sociable and involved. We also decided that we had to straighten out his burial wishes; our mother was buried in New York, where the adjacent plot was reserved for him, but he had mentioned cremation a while back, which appeared to be out of character.

"Dad, we are both very happy with how well things are going with you here in Chicago," I started as we comfortably sat next to him. "But you know that something sudden and terrible could happen, like it happened to Mommy and could have happened to you when you had your surgery." He nodded with the slight welling of tears as often happened when we talked about our late mother's illness, even though almost eight years have passed. "We want to know what it is you would like us to do should you become ill in a way that you cannot make decisions for yourself and it is unlikely that you will improve."

"I trust you to decide for me," he responded. "You have been very good to me and your decisions have been good, even the one to move to Chicago." Although that was nice to hear again, it was not what we needed at this time. There was no question for any of us that he never could have managed by himself in our family home in Brooklyn. It had become rundown for lack of maintenance — he had refused any outside help, a phenomenon that I often see in my own clinical geriatric practice in older people who fiercely protect their privacy and independence.

"Yes, we know that you have designated us as your power of attorney, but we want to know that if we have to make decisions, they will be the ones that we think you would want us to make," we replied.

I continued: "If, for example, you have a stroke or develop Alzheimer's and can no longer communicate reasonably well, enjoy ordinary things like food, be able to get up and about, listen to the radio, read the newspaper — even if it is only the *Chicago Tribune* — and things are likely to get only worse, what would you want us to do?"

"Leave me alone," he replied.

"Do you mean not do anything to keep you alive, for example, if you got pneumonia?"

"Yes, that's what I mean, nothing heroic — just let me go in peace."
We looked at each other and felt we were clear about what he meant.

"Now what about *when* you die, where do you want to be buried and why did you once say to Diti you wanted to be cremated?"

He smiled and said, "I don't want to be a burden to anyone and cremation is easy."

"But it really isn't what we would normally do because of our Jewish heritage and culture, so don't worry about being a bother to us," Diti answered.

We then looked at the pros and cons of his being buried in Chicago while my mother's grave was in New York. "The cemetery in New York is the one from our community, Eyshoshuk, in Lithuania, and it is befitting that you and Mommy be buried there as part of our historical heritage," I said.

"But who will come and visit us and pay tribute?" he asked.

This was clearly an important issue for him, which was interesting, as he generally was not one for symbolism or ritual. He was usually very empirical, having been a respected engineer in the United States Department of Defence. Now he was talking about a strong symbolic value.

My sister replied, "We'll just make it our business to come and visit as part of a weekend in New York."

And I followed up with a quip: "And then, after the cemetery visit, we'll celebrate the two of you as our most wonderful parents and your legacy to us and your grandchildren by going out to eat Chinese food, which has always been a way we celebrated important family events."

We all had a good laugh, and it was agreed.

There was a sense of relief among all of us, now that those important issues were addressed. We agreed that the talk was very helpful and settled some important questions that we might have to struggle with at some time in the future.

This personal experience was partially the result of my repeated professional involvement with situations in which families have not adequately discussed or explored the values and wishes of those for whom they will be responsible. They often struggle with the decisions and feel guilty when a difficult choice is made. It is often very painful for families to make difficult decisions, even with the help of health care staff.

Diti and I, both health care professionals, struggled with the decisions as they related to our mother, so we know that open discussions when there is no crisis might help to clear the air. The goal for us was to achieve a comfort level so that when there is a difficult challenge it can be addressed with warmth, love, and the security that our choices reflect previously expressed values and wishes. Discussions like the one we had with our father do not make such difficult decisions easy, but it makes them easier to live with after the fact.

Sometimes there is a need for a sense of closure as one moves forward on life's journey. I had such an opportunity some time after I had the discussion with my father and Diti. It was the 2004 March break. I had not had a chance to visit my best friend who lived in Manhattan since my father had moved to Chicago from New York. He had helped us pack up the house after my father moved and had been a very close part of our family during my university days and thereafter. The March school break was coming up, and I decided to make a short visit to New York and take my fourteen-year-old son, Eytan, with me, as he had a camp friend in New York and had expressed an interest in visiting her. Now we were in New York for the long weekend.

We were staying at my best friend's upper west side apartment in Manhattan, a great place from which to undertake our daily activities. In addition to walking the streets and doing some shopping, with the main focus on my son's love of rock music, we had short visits with two cousins, one the daughter of my father's youngest sibling (his sister, with whom I had been very close as a child). It was she who had taken me to many of the shows and outings that entranced me as a child and she has always been very dear to me. The other was the daughter of one of my father's brothers, who was famous for his sense of humour, with an endless array of stories and jokes, which would be used to entertain me and my cousins during family gatherings.

On the last day of our trip we agreed to combine a visit with Ellis Island, the entry point of my grandparents from their native Lithuania and Russia at the beginning of the twentieth century, with a visit to Brighton Beach in Brooklyn, where I spent my childhood and from where my father had been moved to Chicago. The museum on Ellis Island is tasteful and moving and resonated strongly in me as I recognized the street scenes of the immigrant neighbourhoods of lower east side New York and the garment district sweatshops that I had heard about in great detail from my seamstress maternal grandmother. Eytan and his sister, Talia, had heard many stories from me about their maternal great-grandmother (my bubby) and had seen some old pictures of her that I retrieved from my parents' home when we emptied it after my father moved to Chicago. As we sailed past the Statue of Liberty on the way back to the dock, I imagined what it must have been like to enter New York's harbour for those millions of immigrants and refugees who had to pass through Ellis Island before entering the country.

We got on the subway and took it to Atlantic Avenue, to change to the B train to Brighton Beach. On the station I explained to Eytan that this was the place I had arrived at each day for three years while I attended Brooklyn Technical High School, one of the special schools in New York that prepared students for entry into science and engineering, which had been my career plan prior to my decision to study medicine. The small blue and white tiles on the station walls looked exactly the same as they had in the mid-1950s when I waited with my arms full of books to return to Brighton Beach, which was the last stop on that subway line. From the train windows I pointed to Cunningham Junior High School, where the new curriculum at the time had required boys and girls to learn typing, performing the repetitive exercises on heavy Underwood typewriters. It was probably the single most useful course I ever took in my educational career, one that prepared me for my university years, where I was one of the few students who did not have to hire a typist for term papers.

We descended the stairs to Brighton Beach Avenue, for much of its length in the shadows of the elevated subway line, which periodically roared above the street. Immediately, it was clear that we had entered another world, one in which mostly Russian immigrants lived and worked and whose stores and restaurants all sported signs written in Russian and sometimes also in English. If this were like Quebec, the language police would be having a field day giving out summonses to shop owners for not highlighting English as the primary language for commerce. As the faces passed, gold crowns on the teeth, a common approach to dental prosthetics in the former Soviet Union, were a common sight. As I pointed out things of note to Eytan, he reminded me that he had actually been in Brighton Beach some years ago to visit his grandfather with me and recognized the neighbourhood, a fact I had forgotten in my plans to show him the place of my roots.

We walked along the boardwalk, away from the famous Coney Island and toward my childhood home. The level of the sand along Brighton Beach had for some reason gradually been elevated until it was almost even with the boardwalk, a sharp contrast to the six- to eight-foot drops from the walkway to the beach that had existed during my childhood years. It was strange to look straight across the sand rather than down at it as we walked along on this crisp, sunny March day. We returned to Brighton Beach Avenue and I had to stop as I saw the sign "Mrs. Stahl's Knishes and Pizza" in bright green and gold letters. The venerable home of the best knishes in the world had been turned into just another fast food eatery, with some attempt to attract those who remembered the delicious aroma and taste of those luscious knishes that could be eaten in the small cramped space in the previous restaurant, bought to be eaten on the street, ordered for home celebrations, or shipped, as the old sign said, "To anywhere in the world" — which it sometimes was. Knishes and pizza — a reflection of the melding of cultures and cuisine in the transformed world of my youth and that of my parents, Roz and Max — today's Brighton Beach.

We walked toward West End Avenue, from where we had moved my father to Chicago. From the time of my last visit about a year ago with my daughter, also to show her for the first time in her life my old neighbourhood, the whole structure of the place of our small, attached bungalow had undergone a dramatic transformation. Parallel to a small medical centre, which had already been built during my father's tenure as a widower in our little bungalow, was another similar medical clinic, and together the two buildings framed the entrance to our little home on both sides so that it appeared to sit back between them, small and insignificant. I pointed out the door to the house, tucked back, having been changed since my father had left it. It was at that moment, while taking a picture to be sent to my father and Diti of the house and the two medical buildings with my son sitting on the curb, that I realized that this visit was likely to be the last time I would ever return to the neighbourhood of my childhood. The era was over, and the memories of my life and those of my parents and sister in this small bungalow where I had studied for high school and college were over. I would tell my father of the transformation during our next phone call and send him the picture. As Eytan and I walked back to the subway, I knew that the memories I shared with my parents and Diti of Brighton Beach would be forever in my soul, and that these memories I shared with my youngest son would be the last additions to the narrative of this chapter of my family's life.

When my father agreed to sell our little house, after he settled in Chicago, both Diti and I were delighted that he had agreed to leave the place of memories with my mother, Roz, and all we had shared during those formative years of our childhood. Saying goodbye now had little emotional impact but did leave a bittersweet sense of history and sharing, which I had just done with Eytan and which allowed him to have a small glimpse into the continuity of the history that he has in common with his immigrant great-grandparents, whom he did not know, and his grandparents, whom he did know but mostly as a very young child and only intermittently, and his father, for whom Brighton Beach was the place that helped to mould who we are.

How and if Eytan and his sister, Talia, will find the connections to all of us as they form their own lives is of course not certain. The distances make it difficult to maintain a sense of intimacy with my father. Eytan and his sister and my older children from my first wife, who knew their grandparents better, will hopefully carry some of their legacy into their own lives in one way or another. I can only hope that the legacy and continuity that I bring to them of my heritage will become part of theirs, and that when the time comes they will be able to understand me and my needs and desires in the same way that I have struggled to understand those of my own parents.

LESSONS LEARNED

The experiences I had with my mother taught me a number of lessons that I have been able to use in helping my father, and my experiences with both of them have taught me lessons that have helped me in my clinical geriatric practice. I can now understand the predicaments of patients and their families, not only from the professional perspective, but also from the personal vantage point.

The experiences with my mother led me to do my best to make sure that I had the conversation with my father about his values and wishes should he fall ill and not be able to make decisions. I realized that sitting down and putting together a written living will was not going to happen, so I told him what I thought the important values were in his life and how I would make decisions if he were to become ill in a manner similar to my mother's experiences. When he confirmed these values and principles, I communicated them to my sister so that we were both party to his wishes and expectations. This proved to be very useful when it came time for him to agree to his cardiac surgery. All he had to do was reiterate that he would want to be "left alone" if he did not make a good recovery, which was enough for us to understand his wishes. The fact that Diti and I had the opportunity to have a face-to-face and heart-to-heart discussion about these issues again a few years later helped us to confirm our understanding of my father's deep-seated wishes and values, which we assume will be of great value when the difficult times we can anticipate in his later years come.

I learned from my mother's illness that children often find it difficult to accept bad outcomes and often take it upon themselves to try to rectify the situation, especially in institutional settings. This is very reasonable and when done properly can lead to some improvements in care. It is useful to understand what clinical options make sense and to try to act on them. It is important not to allow others to make decisions that are very important to a family member. And while well-meaning others may provide advice and input, ultimately it is the family who has to decide what is right. However, once that decision is made, it is important not to revert to "what if" scenarios, but rather to accept that whatever decision was made was the right decision. I use this concept with my patients and families who struggle with decisions. I try to help them understand that there are rarely "right" answers with difficult decisions — they can only do the best they can, and they must live with their decision as the best one they could have made under the circumstances.

One of the important lessons I learned from caring for my father is knowing that timing is often critical in decision-making. It is not possible or proper to force a situation when the parent is not ready for that decision to be made. It becomes counterproductive to keep badgering a parent to make a decision that he or she is not yet prepared to make. I saw this in terms of my father's reluctance to move from his home until it was clear that he was in danger, and also in terms of his hearing aid — when he was ready, that was the only time to act. On the other hand, I also learned and now use in my practice the idea that sometimes waiting until someone is "ready" may be dangerous and result in acting too late. I try to help patients and their families make difficult decisions by outlining the implications of waiting too long to make a necessary move.

Another important lesson I have learned is that you *can* teach an old dog new tricks, meaning that the opportunities to grow and develop can continue at every age. It is not necessarily the case that moving from one's own home to a facility is the beginning of the end; rather, it may be the beginning of a new era of interaction and enjoyment. I have seen this in my practice, but most important, I have now experienced it with my father. He has been transformed from a near-hermit, deteriorating physically and mentally, to a vibrant, active person who participates in social activities, including dancing and exercise programs. To see him greeted by his buddies at the retirement home lunch program was very satisfying for me, as I knew that once again my father Max was a "somebody."

The last and perhaps most important lesson is that helping one's parents can be very challenging, trying, and time-consuming. If possible, share the responsibility with other siblings, and if that is not possible, at least acknowledge and support the siblings who are carrying the main part of the responsibility. I am lucky in having a wonderful sister who is the primary caregiver to my father. I must remind myself how fortunate my father and I are to have her. On the other hand, both my sister and I were fortunate to have had our parents, and caring for them in their later years is a small way of returning to them what they were able to provide for us and of promoting the values that they instilled in us.

A WEEK OF TRAUMA SETS THE STAGE FOR HURT AND HOPE

by Bart Mindszenthy

I finished drafting the first chapter to this book on April 20. Now, only three months later, we're into a new family crisis.

When I started work on *Parenting Your Parents* and Michael Gordon agreed to join with me on this journey, it was my father who was ill and in hospital. The problem? Severe constipation. So severe that I had to get him into the emergency room at North York General Hospital twice — first for a not too successful "extraction," which is a very messy form of "digital digging" into the rectum, and then again for enemas and more digital work.

The second round meant staying in the hospital for three days to ensure his bowel was functioning. Plus, my father needed a catheter inserted into his penis because his bladder was blocked. With all this, he was grumpy, miserable, in pain, and out of it because of the Demerol injections given to relieve the pain. But with his usual will and tenacity, and because he is willing to listen to what needs to be done, he's regained a bit of his health. He's not in great shape, but he keeps pushing along, ever so slowly, and ever so carefully.

Since his hospitalization, my mother has taken a turn for the worse. It's a situation that's been brewing for some weeks. My mother's been like a pot of water on the stove with the heat turned up high — eventually the water boils, and if the pot isn't taken off, the water bubbles over.

And my mother's mind is now boiling.

What follows is a chronicle of the past week. It's self-explanatory. It's all about what happens when a parent is undergoing rapidly advancing dementia that is suspected to be the dreaded Alzheimer's disease. There's nothing nice about any of this. It's painful for all involved, and right now I feel a huge amount of love for both my mother, who's entering the "twilight zone" of her older age, and my father, who will have to witness his wife of nearly six decades change before his non-seeing eyes into someone who will become totally different in the time they have left together.

If there is a hope, it's that in some way we'll manage to work through this dire challenge and be able to help and support my mother, to make her as comfortable as possible, and to somehow let her know how much we love her and care about her well-being. And hopefully my father will be able to cope with the fact that we can't ever go back to where we were: that nothing will be sure or safe or right again in the times ahead.

July 24, 2001

Dementia, my parents' doctor tells me, cuts a broad swath through the mind and behaviour of the elderly. Dementia is a single word that means so little and affects so much. It ranges across a spectrum that goes from pre-dementia, to mild, then moderate, through to severe, and then the end stage. Bottom line: cognitive capabilities decline — memory, judgment, insight, and reason. Which is a nice way of saying that the mind is no longer able to do the work it once did, and that step by step there is a new mindset that is confusing, difficult to accept, and eventually impossible to understand for all those who are in the midst of it.

Dementia means many different things to many people, but what it means most to all of us who have a parent experiencing it is that there is a growing gap between what we used to experience with a parent and what is now happening.

My parents' doctor has given my mother a carefully balanced set of medications to help her cope with her increasingly fragile mental state. She's been tested in just about every imaginable way. A geriatric assessment team has spent time with her twice in the past six months, and then there were the CT scans and the blood work and the neurologist's examination. All of it has resulted in little more than the conclusion that my mother is far more demented than she was six or twelve months ago, and that, in fact, she's now delusional.

This diagnosis is borne out by her most recent allegations that my father — nearing ninety-six — and one of the women who come in to help them (who's in her late thirties) are having a sexual relationship. The accusations started several weeks ago when my mother became agitated because the helper was stroking my father's arm, and it built from there.

Yesterday, my mother claimed that the helper was in bed with my father.

Just today, she maintained that the helper was nude in my father's room, then in bed with him. She also asserted that the helper was stealing things from the house and lying about what medication my mother is taking.

This afternoon, my mother actually physically attacked my father, hitting and slapping him, and tried to hit the helper with her cane.

I talked to my parents at least a dozen times today on the telephone because I'm away. The concern, worry, agony, fear, anger, and love are overwhelming as the stress of the situation courses through me. Each time we talk, I hear the beleaguered voice of my father, weak as it is, straining to be heard, telling me how concerned he is about my mother and how terrible he feels — how her imagination is getting the best of her. He asks how I can help, and I tell him that I just don't know, because I'm way beyond my competency given the situation. He wants me to drive to their house in Toronto, and I ask what that will achieve, and he tells me probably nothing.

When my mother gets on the phone, she's full of venom. Her anger is awesome and overwhelming. She verbally attacks my father: how could he have sexual relations with this woman after so many years of marriage, all through which she's been faithful and so caring of him and me. And how can he deny his transgression? And then my mother sets in on me: how is it possible that I, her son, could possibly question her about what she's seen. How is it possible that I would doubt her word when she's always been there for me over these many years. It's a nasty conversation during which I sometimes lose control and verbally shoot back and sometimes try very hard to give her comfort.

The reason we have so many telephone sessions is that my mother keeps hanging up on me. After one such set of calls, I telephone my parents' doctor and leave a message, asking him to call me as soon as he can. Then, in the next call to my mother, she tells me that I've abandoned her, that I've sided with my father, that I've been brainwashed by others, and that I've fallen to the charms of this helper of theirs as well. Along the way, my mother hurls a host of personal insults that sting and tear into my own mind, to a point where I don't know what to do to help my parents or myself.

Somewhere through these conversations, their doctor returns my call, and I can hear in his voice the concern for both my mother and my father. He does something very special: he tells me he's going to call my mother tonight to talk with her. And he's going to look at whether it might be best to get her admitted into our local hospital's geriatric ward for a break and an assessment.

Later tonight, I talk on the phone again to my parents. My mother is totally illogical. I try very hard to cope and to find some common ground with her. My father sounds even weaker than usual and totally drained, telling me that my mother's mind is confused and that we need to help her. While I agree with him, I don't know what to do or how to do it best.

Rushing through my own mind is a mix of frustration, love, and doubt.

They're old, I tell myself. Very old. What can I do for either and both of them? Then my mother comes on the line, still passionate with her anger and hurt. I try very hard to be calm and cool and loving, and it's a challenge as she again rips into me for being selfish and siding with my father and completely blinded by my hate for her.

I don't know how to handle this. My own personal world is in chaos. On the one hand, I want to reach out and hug my mother and remind her that I'm her son and love her and that I'll take care of her forever. On the other hand, I want to yell at her that she's not dealing with the real world and that her mind's playing tricks on her, pushing her further and further into a false world created by her advancing dementia.

But I've learned enough working on this book to know that to challenge her right now would be wrong and of no use. My mother is off into another dimension and the best I can do is try to listen, absorb the hurt, and see if I can in some way generate a calming effect on her. And I fail at this. I'm into new territory I don't know how to manage.

Later that evening, my partner, Gail, provides an excellent reality check by asking me a series of questions over a subdued dinner.

What do I think I can really do for my mother by being logical when she's not? When did my mother begin to show signs of behaving this way? What did my father or I do to help her in the past? How much of this load do I think I can carry, and for how long? How long do I think my parents can manage this family crisis? The truth is that I don't know the answers to any of Gail's questions.

What I do know is that I'm mentally and emotionally and physically drained by what's happened this long day. Late into the night, I'm conscious and worried about my mother and my father, hoping that both can and will sleep deep and well into tomorrow so that we might move on and get this mess behind us.

JULY 25, 2001

During the night, my mother stayed in my father's bed and talked all night. Once she hit him again, and another helper who spends nights with them tried to restrain her. The helper tells me that both of them are exhausted, yet my mother continues to verbally badger my father, like a tape running over and over again. I hear this when she calls to tell me I'd better come to help. We're staying at our country home for a few weeks, with me going into town every couple of days to check on them, shop for food they need, and get our mail. Gail also stopped by when she was in town last week.

So I rush to the city, and in the process I manage to get a hefty speeding ticket. En route I try to call my parents' geriatric specialist but can't get through. I leave an urgent message, which is never returned. Then I call their family doctor, who calls back quickly. I tell him what's happened and that my mother has apparently stopped taking her pills; it seems she's claiming that she doesn't know what she's taking or why, and so she's not taking anything. He urges me to bring her into the hospital — where he'll be later in the day — and says that it would be a good idea to keep her in for a couple of days to do assessments and get her on her medication. Plus, he says, this would give my father a rest. He also tells me that if I can't get her to come with me, I might have to ask for assistance from the police.

When I get to my parents' house, my mother is still going on about my father and his alleged infidelity. She then takes some well-aimed verbal shots at me. I ask her several times to come with me to the hospital, and she refuses. It's exasperating. Then, suddenly, she agrees to come. She dresses, and then when she's ready and eating their usual very late breakfast, she tells me she's not coming after all — that there's nothing wrong with her if people would just leave her alone. Throughout, she keeps talking in a totally disjointed way — zigging this way and then zagging that way in her train of thought.

And there's a new behaviour I notice for the first time: every time I look at my father, or I go and do something in another room, or I touch something that's hers, my mother immediately wants to know what I'm doing and if I'm taking something that's hers. Repeatedly she talks about people stealing things from her or from their house. She alleges that we're all in collusion against her. And, worst for me to hear, she tells me over and over that I'm a total disappointment because I'm working against her, believing others and not her. My mother demands to know how I could have changed so much for the worse and who is influencing me to turn against her.

And on and on it goes. And like playing spin the bottle or the roulette wheel, where it stops, no one knows. But it doesn't stop at all. It just changes directions, her mind obviously churning myriad confused thoughts.

On the front porch of their house, where my mother can't hear us, I ask my father what he would like me to do, because it's clear that there's no way she'll voluntarily come with me to the hospital. We discuss options, and I tell him of my concern for both his well-being and hers.

He thinks about it, then says that calling the police to take her to the hospital would probably do more immediate harm than if we tried to get her to a calmer state for a day or two and then try again. I'm not convinced.

I ask him again to consider the pressure on him and on all of us. But he's thought about it and stands by his decision.

I acquiesce because I respect his mind, and because he is a psychologist by training. I know he's old, but my father is mentally strong, even if physically very weak.

When we go back in, my mother asks if my father and I remember that a while ago we all stood in the hallway, made the peace sign, and shook hands to agree that we'll all be all right again. I reply that didn't happen at all. My father agrees with me. And my mother immediately starts on another harangue about how we're conspiring to work against her. A thought flashes through my mind — something Michael told me in one of our early meetings. He'd said that sometimes, when an older person is demented and delusional, if she or he believes something that's not real but also not harmful, it might be all right to let it be real. So I backtrack and tell my mother I don't mean it didn't happen, only that I don't remember. And I propel my father into the kitchen and whisper to him that he should remember we shook hands and agreed, which is precisely what he does as he walks back into the living room. My mother looks victorious; she tells me that this is a good example of my own forgetfulness and confusion. We got a tiny step ahead for the moment, although it wasn't easy.

Moments later, she starts again about why and how I'm not being supportive of her. I manage to inject into her newest outpouring of confused thoughts that I've got some errands to do and that I'll be back later.

So I leave them for a few hours to get our mail, stop for a brief meeting, and do some grocery shopping for them. Along the way, my twenty-three-year-old daughter, Andrea, calls me on the cell phone, wanting to know how I am and how her grandparents are and to tell me about what she's doing. I give her a fast update. She's shaken by her grandmother's decline and says she's going to call them and then call me back.

Andrea calls me back some ten minutes later to report that her grandmother indeed sounds very confused. She tells me that she's very worried by what she's heard and scared by what her grandmother said, which was, in essence, that things are not right and that I'm one of the main causes. Andrea also talked to her grandfather and told him she understands how traumatic this is for all of them, especially for him.

Andrea, by the way, is in her final year at university studying neuropsychology.

She asks if she should come to help. I'm moved and thank her, but recommend that there's nothing she can do to help right now.

When I return from errands and shopping, my parents are having supper. My mother tells me that while I was away, she and my father had a good talk and that they've agreed to put all this behind them, not talk about it any more, and get on with their lives. I'm delighted, relieved, and hopeful that perhaps we might have gotten over this family crisis. I have a bit to eat with them. Then my mother says we need to have a discussion about how I feel. I tell her that there's nothing to discuss; if they've agreed to put "this" behind them, that's all I care about. I suggest that we should never talk about it again, but it's clear my mother wants to do just that.

By now I'm tired and thinking about the drive ahead. So I tell her that I'm concerned for both of them, and that for the sake of all of us, we should agree not to talk about this any more.

We all agree, and I leave.

And so another intense episode passes. Where this leads, I don't know. I only know I'm very tired. I know I'm watching and experiencing another level of descent into the vortex of dementia and all the challenges it's presenting. How we'll deal with it is a mystery to me. What I do know is that I'm afraid for both my mother and my father — for what each must cope with while we find a way forward and for the strength they will need to face the next hurdle.

July 26, 2001

The phone rings early afternoon. In his strained, reedy voice, my father tells me my mother is again on a verbal binge. She's still stuck in the "how-could-you-do-this-to-me" mode, and he asks me to come back from the country where I'm working on this book to help. I honestly don't want to. I'm terrified of where this is leading.

I can hear my mother in the background yelling at my father to give her the phone, and when he keeps talking to me, I hear her attack him.

It's terrifying. She comes on the line and continues her rant about my father's infidelity, about how I don't seem to care, and about her personal hurt and shame. This goes on for a few minutes, and then my father is back on, asking when I can be there. Although I had dedicated this day to writing, I tell him I'll come as soon as possible, but that I need to try to reach their family physician first. I try, but he's not in. I call the geriatric clinic and talk to one of the staff who a month ago spent time with my parents in their home. She's very understanding and gives me some good options for getting immediate help. The best is to contact something called the Mobile Crisis Team, and that's what I do first.

The woman who answers the phone at the Mobile Crisis Team is wonderful, understanding, and ready to help once I explain the state of affairs. Heidi tells me a team can be at my parents' house when I get there, and that if they determine there is danger to my mother or father, they'll arrange to have my mother taken to the hospital, even if it means calling in the police. I call to tell my father I'm on my way, then I change, jump in the car, and head off.

When I'm about half an hour away from my parents', I call Heidi back. This time I get her partner, Leslie, who explains that they're on the way to another emergency visit, but to call when I get to my parents' house and they'll come as soon as possible.

I get to my parents' house and call Heidi and Leslie on the cell phone while sitting in the car in the driveway. They're busy helping someone else, but they tell me that as soon as they're done — and they're not too far away — they'll come to see us.

I take a deep breath and knock on my parents' front door. My father opens it, looking gaunt and drained. My mother is sitting in her usual chair in the living room. When she sees me, she begins to explain intensely all the wrongs done to her by this conspiracy of people. We talk, argue, back off, start talking some more, and keep going in circles that leave none of us feeling any better. This goes on for an hour.

We continue at the kitchen table while we eat dinner. Then my cell phone rings: it's Leslie to say they're out in front of the house, and I tell them they're needed. When they come in, Heidi takes the lead and she's wonderful: relaxed, easygoing, and non-confrontational. My mother, who for some time has been so vocal and emotional, is suddenly the epitome of sweetness and reason. I'm amazed by the transformation. Meanwhile, Heidi just keeps talking and asking questions, and each time my mother gets her back up, Heidi backs down to give my mother more comfort space. For example, when Heidi first asks about what medications she's taking, my mother won't tell, yet five minutes later, she's showing Heidi all her bottles of pills. So it goes for the better part of half an hour, until Heidi asks my mother a series of questions that somehow gets my mother to drop the facade and revert to her behaviour of the past weeks. She becomes more belligerent and aggressive and keeps questioning why anyone would possibly want to doubt her version of reality.

After also asking my father some questions, Heidi thanks my parents for their time and says goodbye and signals me to follow her out, where, on the front porch, Leslie is concluding a cell phone conversation with another family in distress. As we stand in the driveway, Heidi tells me they can't call the police or anyone else to take my mother into the hospital, because while they believe my mother is delusional and a danger to herself and my father — and even me — there's no observed behaviour to support that contention.

So they give me more options. One is to have my parents' family doctor make a house call and convince my mother to go into the hospital for an assessment. Another is to go to a justice of the peace and plead my case for a ruling that would allow my mother to be forcefully taken to a hospital for an assessment and treatment plan. And a third is to get my parents' family doctor or the geriatric specialist to sign a "Form One" and admit her to the geriatric psychiatric section at the local hospital for seventy-two hours of assessment and treatment.

Some choices. I don't want any of them. Each is plagued with personal and family danger. This is not where I want to be. No matter what I do, I realize, I'm going to hurt someone — my mother, my father, me, my children, my partner, my parents' few remaining friends — which means that as far as my mother is concerned, I'm going to be the villain. That's a lot of weight to carry, I think. But then again, I realize that it's not like I have many workable choices. As my friend and colleague Harvey Silver, an organizational psychologist, likes to remind one and all, we always have choices; we just need to consider them and decide, since even doing nothing is a choice we make.

When I go back in to talk to my parents again, I convince my mother to see the geriatric specialist, whom they'd seen some six months ago. I ask her if she'd come with me to see him so we can talk about what medications she should be taking and to review how she's doing.

My mother says she'll come as long as we can also go have a cappuccino together afterward, and I agree. I feel like a traitor, a Judas, because I've already arranged the appointment with the doctor, and I know he'll give her two choices: to voluntarily go straight to the hospital or to have them sign a Form One and be taken in.

It's on that note that I head for my house in the city to get some sleep. I'm depressed, tired, and confused; I tell myself I'm doing the right thing and then second-guess myself the next moment. I have this ongoing debate in my head about what to do and recognize that in this case, I simply must get her the kind of help she needs, because we're all self-destructing the way things are going.

JULY 27, 2001

I call the doctor's office in the morning and talk with the woman who's been my contact and who's met my parents. We discuss the options again, and she assures me that, given her own assessment of my parents about a month ago, we must get my mother into the hospital.

I call my mother and tell her she has to get up and get ready for a 10:45 a.m. session with the doctor and that she should bring all her medications. Then I get ready, drive to my parents' home, and collect my mother and her five bottles of pills. She's agitated, confused, and confusing.

The doctor's office is only a five-minute drive, and we get there on time, and then — what else is new? — we wait. He's running behind.

Eventually, he comes to get us and take us to his office. He's not the epitome of warmth and charisma, but he's very good at what he does.

So it's a tense meeting right from the get-go. He spends some minutes looking at what's now become a rather thick file and asks her some questions, many of which my mother doesn't understand; some, neither do I, but I translate as best I can.

The long and short of it is that the doctor asks her to voluntarily check into the hospital immediately. My mother tells him there's nothing wrong with her, and that, no, she won't do that. Then he tells her that if she won't agree to go with me to the hospital, he'll have to sign the Form One and have the police take her there. My mother is clearly devastated, but says, no, she won't go. She looks at me and asks how I could do this to her — her only child, turning on her like this. And on it goes for another five minutes, when the doctor asks us to wait in the reception area.

My mother and I sit there, and for the better part of an hour she assaults me with a host of allegations about my memory, my behaviour, my lifestyle, and everything else she can think of. Added to it all are various threats about what she'll do to me and my reputation and threats about how my father will die if I go through with this. She argues, she pleads, and she verbally attacks me as we sit there; she stops people walking by and asks for help, and she eventually says she wants nothing to do with me ever again and gets up and moves four seats away from me.

I'm in a living real-time hell — as I know she must be. I keep telling her this is not something I want to see happen, or like, but that there just isn't any other choice. We argue, and we ignore each other.

Finally, a squad car with two police officers arrives. They walk over to us and talk with my mother, asking her to come with them. She says she won't. But they are very gentle and caring and amazingly patient.

They kid with her, and they compliment her, and eventually they get her to stand up and head for the door. Meanwhile, several staff are looking on, and some of them even come by and whisper to me that I mustn't take this personally and that I'm doing the right thing.

I'm almost in tears. This is so hurtful and painful. It's real and happening, and it shouldn't be. I feel a huge amount of love and sorrow and anxiety and hurt. It's like the morning my marriage died and I watched the faces of my children as I left. It's one of those experiences that stay with me for a lifetime. All I know is that I don't want to be here, to be in this scene. However, it's still better happening this way, here, and not in my parents' home with my father there.

The police officers are considerate yet again. They suggest that my mother ride in my car rather than in the patrol car. My mother tells them I'm not her son anymore, and she doesn't care. But in the end she sits in the front seat beside me, with one of the officers in the back seat and the other in the patrol car following. While my mother tells me that I'm the bane of her life and a worthless son she never wants to see again, I, for some crazy reason, become very conscious of driving right at the speed limit and using my turn signal at every turn we make. And so we get to the hospital emergency room, which is flooded with people.

While the officers help my mother check in, I rush back to my parents' house to tell my father what is happening. He sits in stunned, sad silence. He sighs deeply several times. His quivering hands are clutched together, and he looks at me with such sorrow that I want to cry again.

I ask him: what else could we do? I ask him: isn't this going to help my mother — his wife of fifty-eight years — get the help she needs? Won't this give him a break from the tension that's been hanging smog-like in their house for the past weeks? My father acknowledges that it's the right thing but says it hurts, and I see the quiver of his lips for the first time in my life. And I know how much pain he also is experiencing at this moment. He wants to know how long she'll be in the hospital, and I tell him I don't know, even though I do know it's at least four days. But I don't want to make him feel even worse. I keep telling him that it's for the best, and he just nods and tells me that's probably right.

I rush back to the emergency room reception area and wait there with my mother for two hours. The police officers are helpful and considerate beyond anything I'd have expected. Finally, my mother's name is called, and we're taken to a cubicle in the treatment area. That's where we'll spend the next six hours, locked in verbal combat. I don't want to argue; I keep telling my mother that we're here to get her the help she needs, and she keeps telling me that she's fine. We go around and around in circles of complex and confusing dialogue. A few times I manage to get out and call my father to give him an update, and to call my partner, Gail, to tell her what's going on.

My mother has now decided that this is a jail or prison of some kind. I keep assuring her it's not. And just to add to the drama and trauma of this event, the police arrive with a stocky, barrel-chested man in leg shackles and handcuffs, who's plunked on a bed two cubicles down from where we're sitting. Of course, this adds more fuel to my mother's mental fire. Now we are in a prison, and we're just waiting for her cell to be cleared. And so it goes. We talk nicely, we talk passionately, and we argue.

A woman who's been there for almost twenty-four hours with her aging ill mother waiting for a bed comes by, and we strike up a conversation, and this gives me a chance to run out and find a sandwich and juice for my mother and me to share.

Time passes. Finally, two women arrive. They introduce themselves, and I can't remember the name of either. They tell us they're the crisis team. They sit and talk with my mother for about three-quarters of an hour, asking her a lot of questions. My mother responds and does quite well with her broken English. I urge her to tell them what she's most upset about, and she does: about my father's affair with their helper, and what a shame this is, and how terrible it all is, and how she's over that now, but how it hurts. The two women thank my mother for her time and tell her that soon she'll be moved upstairs.

Then we're alone again for another hour. My mother gives me several ultimatums that are essentially the same: get her out of here and take her home so she can care for my father, or he'll probably die.

Yet another hour passes and finally a cheerful orderly arrives with a wheelchair, only to discover we've already got one. So he picks ours and helps my mother into it, while she continues to tell me I've got one final chance to repent and relent and take her home. I keep telling her that I can't do anything right now and that we've got to get her the help she needs.

Upstairs, on the seventh floor, we are buzzed into the geriatric psychiatry wing. I read the sign and watch the procedure, and I'm on the edge of tears again. I can't believe I'm doing this: that my mother is here and so am I.

A bubbly nurse emerges from the locked nursing station and we wheel my mother into a private room with a large glass window in the door and its own bathroom. Then we tour the self-contained area while some woman with an accent almost as good as my mother's sings in a loud voice somewhere down the hall. By the time we get to the communal dining room, hearing yet a few other people yelling and seeing others walking up and down the hallway, I keep thinking about the book and amazing movie *One Flew Over the Cuckoo's Nest*. I just can't believe we're here, or that we have to be here. There is something totally terrifying about this, and yet I honestly believe that if we're to save my parents' lives for a while longer, this is what we must do.

Back in my mother's room — her cell, as she calls it — I try to get her as comfortable as possible. She's cold, and we get some extra covers, but the fact is hospitals are cold all of the time, and for the elderly this is another discomfort.

I tell her I'll bring her a bathrobe, some other clothes, and her toiletries. This is of small consolation to my mother. She wants to know again why I did this to her and how long she has to stay in this terrible place, which, I must admit, it is. She reminds me that I betrayed her and pledges that she won't last more than a day here. She says again that by doing this to her I'm killing her and my father, who can't last on his own.

There's not much I can say. I'm hurting. I feel guilty. I'm tired. I'm scared. I'm fifty-five years old and would much rather crawl in my mother's arms so we can just hug each other. Instead, I help her change into hospital garb and get her into the bed, and I assure her I'll be back in the morning. I leave, and I want to die of fear and shame.

I go back to my parents' house and sit in the kitchen with my father, who's nursing a Scotch and looking so pale and so sad that I don't know what to do or say. We sit there awhile in silence, and I start telling him that things will be all right. I see that he's about to cry — this father of mine who's close to ninety-six years of age and who's always managed his emotions with perfection. Finally, he agrees that my mother needs the attention and care she'll get at the hospital. He tells me that he knows this is right, but that it's still so very traumatic.

We sit there at the kitchen table and chat for a while. He's also very tired. I go and find a small suitcase and pack up clothes and toiletries for my mother, and when I'm done, I tell him to get some sleep. We agree I'll go see her in the morning and take him in to see her in the early afternoon.

And so we hug and part and I drive to the house in the city, feeling totally empty inside.

July 28, 2001

I get to the hospital late morning after a night of restless sleep. I'm tired and stressed. I'm afraid of what condition my mother will be in when I get there. En route, I stop to buy her a sweatsuit, which I think will be comfortable and warm. I buy myself a muffin in the hospital lobby because I'm very hungry. And up I go — back to that seventh-floor prison. I buzz. I'm admitted. I go to the nursing station and meet and talk with the nurse who's looking after my mother and she is very nice and helpful.

When she looks at what I have brought, she tells me I can't give my mother any nightgowns, only the bathrobes. I can't give her the sweatsuit, but I can give her the toiletries kit, and yes, I was smart to take out the razor blades and substitute one of my electric shavers. She says that my mother's doing all right, but that she's somewhat delusional.

My mother is sitting on the bed. She wants to know if I've come to take her home. No, I tell her, not yet, because they have to do some tests.

She gets angry. She wants to know why more tests are needed. She says that she's peeing and pooping quite well and she wants to go home. And, she tells me, a doctor came in to see her and talk with her and he also said she was doing really well. I show her what I have brought — the bathrobes, socks, toiletries, slippers, and a few other things. Meanwhile, I dig out the muffin and share it with her while I listen to her tell me what a horrible night she's had.

We spend an hour talking, with my mother seeming more subdued but still very angry with me. I help her into the bathroom and onto the toilet and wait outside until she's done, and then I help her get organized again and into a chair when her lunch arrives. Then she starts again to verbally attack me for what I've done to her, and my personal guilt monitor soars at once. While I feel huge pity for my mother, concurrently there is also a sense of anger for these continuing attacks, and I try very hard to control my emotions and my tongue so I don't say something I'll regret and in the process exacerbate an already fragile situation. So I tell her I'm going to get my father to bring him for a visit.

When I wheel him into her room an hour later, she's instantly in tears. He slowly gets out of the wheelchair and she slowly stands, and they hug and kiss. It's both heartwarming and heartbreaking to watch.

I stay a bit, then leave them to run some errands. When I return, they're sitting and talking as quietly as is possible for two people who are hard of hearing.

We all chat a while longer and I can see that my father is tiring, so I suggest we leave. There are a lot more tears and hugs and kisses before I wheel him back to the car and drive him home and then head back to the country myself.

I'm really, truly tired, both physically and mentally. I've been dashing to their home most days for several weeks and always spending way more time than I'd anticipated. I'm behind in my client work. And I'm way behind on my parts of this book. Michael is being highly understanding and supportive because he knows what I'm going through on both the personal and professional level. However, I need to get my mind in gear, and it's difficult.

Tonight, I call my daughter Andrea and ask her and her wonderful partner if they'd give me a day off and go see my father tomorrow and take him to visit my mother. They say they're pleased to do so, and that relieves me.

July 29, 2001

It's amazing how tired I am. I worked for a couple of hours on this chronicle of events last night and then fell into bed and woke up not long before noon. I walk around, numb and dumb, for an hour and decide that today for a few hours I need to do mindless work around the property, so I paint things and glue things and change some light fixtures and move slowly. I even have a short nap late in the afternoon.

Through it all, I am mulling over the events of the past days, relating them to the past months, and trying to fit those all into the past years.

I try to figure out if there is a pattern we missed, or if there is some special event that may be important. I think there are some pieces that loosely fit, but I realize that I'm just speculating.

Then my father calls to say that he, Andrea, and Julian had a good visit with my mother and that she seems much calmer overall, and that he misses her and would like her back at home. He also asks me to call her, which I was planning on doing anyway, and see what I think. Then my daughter calls to tell me that her grandmother was in pretty good shape from all she could see and hear. This is heartening news.

I call the geriatric psychiatry wing nursing station and ask how I can speak to my mother. There is one patient phone and it's busy, so the nurse takes pity on me and gets my mother to her phone so we can talk for a few minutes. She actually does sound much more subdued and generally calmer. I feel good about that, although part of me is worried that this may be just a false positive signal and that more bad things may come sooner than later. But even given that cautionary thought, I want to believe that we're on the path to some kind of stable footing for the good of all of us.

JULY 30, 2001

Early this afternoon, my mother's in-hospital doctor calls. He asks me several questions about how I see her state of mind and general condition now compared to last week and suggests we meet tomorrow morning. He tells me that he thinks she might be able to go home the next day or so.

I call my father with this news, and I can sense him perking up right over the phone line. I ask him to think about what's best for him and for her and tell him I'll pick him up in a few hours.

Driving into the city, I reflect on the complexity of being a family member dealing with a loved one who's demented. It's sort of like a Catch-22. If my mother thinks something that isn't real is real, how do we deal with that? My experience so far is that it's a no-win debate.

The people who are watching her witness all sorts of times she's imagined things. There are myriad instances when my mother simply denies reality and clings with a passion to her point of view. My father and I have talked about this many times during these past months, and he just shakes his head and tells me sometimes we simply have to let go and let her reality be the one we go with. This troubles me greatly.

Where do you draw the line? How do we help our parents find the truth so that we can deal with it? Yet as Michael has said to me, sometimes if the reality of a demented person isn't hurtful, maybe it's best to let it be — to let it be their reality. If a demented person with Alzheimer's believes it's Tuesday, for example, but really it's Wednesday, and in the greater scheme of life that doesn't matter, then perhaps that's how we should leave it. I see the sense in all of this, but it's still hard to practise.

By the time I think about all this and end up nowhere, I'm at my parents' house to take my father to see my mother. Today she's sitting in her chair in her room, and she lights up like a birthday candle when I wheel him in. The hugs and kisses are sincere and laden with overwhelming affection. Again, I sit around and talk for a little while and then leave to let them have time alone. And again, when I return, my mother tells me that there's nothing wrong with her mind and demands to know why I am subjecting her to this humiliation and personal pain.

Even as she says this, she's confusing things and alleging things that just aren't so. But it is evident that she is much calmer overall, and that's somewhat reassuring.

She wants to know how long she has to stay. She explains that she met the doctor today and that he said she looked really well and all her tests were fine, and that it was up to me to get her home. We talk around this one for a little while, and my father injects that we should wait and see what the doctor has to say, and that being in the hospital is actually good for my mother, since it gives her a much-needed period of rest.

As I drive my father home, I ask him if he's really comfortable with the possibility of my mother coming home tomorrow. Can he cope? Will she cope? Will those who help them cope? I explain that I'm not just tired, but I need to do my work, and work on this book, and that while I love them dearly, I can't stop my world all the time to help, as selfish as that may seem to him. He understands and says that if the medications are right, it all should work out for the best. For how long, I ask, and he responds that the next critical stage will be another traumatic event that my mother will see as a threat to any one of us, but especially to herself.

He's very logical in his thinking, and I respect his mind.

So we part, and I tell him I'll either be reporting after seeing the doctor, or be bringing my mother home. He says he hopes I'll be bringing her home now that he's rested and ready. He smiles and tells me that this part of his life sure isn't what he expected it to be.

July 31, 2001

This morning I get to the hospital early and wait for the resident psychiatric doctor at the nursing station. I sit around for a while and then look into my mother's room. She's sitting on the bed, sorting through some clothes. My strategy had been to avoid my mother and see the doctor, because I was frankly afraid of what I'd find or how things would go with her. But she looks up about the same time as I'm looking in, and she smiles and calls for me. I go in and kiss her, and she's so happy for the moment. Then she tells me that even though she's totally fine, she was told she couldn't go home today. I say that as far as I know, she maybe can go home today, but that I'm waiting and watching for the doctor to arrive and I don't want to miss him.

My mother and I have this disjointed conversation that covers how bad the nurses are to how badly she slept to how good the food is to how well she slept to how some spies are being kept down the hall to how nice the nurses are, all in one long outpouring. But she is much calmer, and her eyes are clearer and more focused.

After a few minutes, I tell her that I should go back in the hall to wait for the doctor, and she agrees, and that's what I do.

The doctor arrives in a flurry of energy and kindly intensity. After we shake hands he tells me to follow him to someone's office way down the hall. My mother sees this and calls out to me, tells me to help her get home, and I assure her that's utmost on my agenda.

In the office we meet with a really gentle and caring nurse and a social worker. We spend forty-five minutes talking about my mother's condition, what safeguards she needs, how we need to deal with her condition, and what medications she will require. I learn that after all the many tests these past many months, and through a process of elimination, they have diagnosed my mother with Alzheimer's. She's at about mid-point, which is bad, I know, from reading the material Michael has given me and from the conversations he and I have had.

In fact, the doctor tells me, most people in the same condition are institutionalized, but because my parents have care in the home and because my mother could respond to medications, her remaining at home is a viable option.

Then I collect my mother so she can talk with him for a few minutes as he explains the medications he's assigned for her. I want him to do that to avoid her suggesting again that medicines are sent to her without explanation.

The doctor also asks my mother how she is doing, and she assures him that she feels fine and that she appreciates the help she's been given, and how she's done so well in demonstrating her mental agility through all the tests she's taken. It's a sad moment for me. Almost as an afterthought — but a good one — the doctor suggests that he give my mother an overnight pass and that we come back tomorrow for a short meeting to see how my mother's doing before she's discharged. We all agree.

Back in her room, we pack her things and wait for the nurse to bring the medications my mother needs to take until her return visit. My mother is suspicious, wondering if they will really let her leave now or if they are going to keep her again when we come back tomorrow. I assure her that everything will be just fine.

With overnight bag in hand and pill packets in my pocket, we leave the wing, but only after a long battle with the armed door, because the staff person presses the wrong button and the door won't open, which reinforces my mother's impression that she's been confined in a jail of some kind. And we head home. Along the way, we stop at a convenience store and I get a few cans of her favourite soft drink. My motive is to use my cell phone while I'm in the store to call my father and alert him about my mother's condition and what that requires of all of us.

When we arrive at my parents' house, my father is at the front door, all smiles, standing wobbly, but proud and happy. My mother works her way up the front porch steps, across the porch, and they hug and kiss.

Another heart-melting moment for me, as surely it is for them.

For the next hour, we talk about my mother's experiences in the hospital, which she still thinks was a prison of some kind with spies, the too-cold air conditioning, the lack of help, the tests, and on and on. My mother says things that surprise and stun me, but I think I've learned to accept her world without challenge and debate. It's not easy, or realistic, or practical, but very necessary. As Michael and the psychiatric doctor both have said to me, it's important not to agitate a demented person, because that only serves as a trigger to another, more intense, irrational reaction.

On my drive home, I think about how we baby boomers all over are facing the same kind of crisis. We're worrying about our children and we're needing to care for our parents. Some call it the sandwich generation. Whatever you call it, the fact is that we're stuck carrying a lot of baggage, a lot of worry, and a whole lot of responsibility. And guess what? It's not fun.

But then again, maybe it's not a crisis at all. Maybe it's just one more rock to roll up the hill as Sisyphus did in Greek mythology: a test of ourselves and our patience and endurance and commitment and the depth of our love for family. And if we're to pass that test, we've got to be a bit selfish. We've got to recognize that we won't be able to help our aging parents or our children if we don't take time out for ourselves. Easier said than done, yes, but critically important. As I talk and work with doctors and nurses and caregivers who are much more experienced and wiser than I am, they have one clear and consistent message: I'm the one who's delivering for them, and if I can't, it won't happen.

So what does that mean? It means, quite simply, that if I drop the ball, it's game over for all of us, because I'll be of no use to anyone, and my parents won't get the level and range of help they need and deserve. And I will certainly drop the ball if I get too stressed out or, worse, sick. Michael has talked a lot about the need to bear this in mind and to deal with it.

As I think about this, it seems to me that for those of us who, by design or default, end up as primary caregivers to our parents there are three serious challenges to face: managing the physical demands of time and stress; managing the mental drain of focusing so hard on their needs; and managing the frustration and guilt we feel as matters worsen.

To face the physical demands we have to arrange our priorities in such a way that we don't compromise the other parts of our lives. From my own experience in the past half-year especially, it's obvious that if we take on the task of helping our parents, the demands for time and attention will grow rapidly. In order not to jeopardize our other family commitments and our vocational expectations, we have to create some level of balance and set priorities. For example, I've talked to all three of my children and explained that right now I'm in a very difficult and demanding time with their grandparents, and so, for a while at least, they need to understand that I'll have less time for them. I have explained that this doesn't reflect a lack of love for them, but that it's a balancing act I hope they understand. I think they do.

On the work side, it's a matter of ensuring "the job" gets done. In my case, I'm fortunate that we have our own business and can juggle client work between Gail and me. It's also fortunate that as I'm deep into this especially trying time, we're not that busy — although that's a double-edged sword, because not being very busy also means not generating the level of income we need. Others I know who are engulfed in parental caregiving and who work tell me that managing their work life has become very difficult, as they need to ask for more and more time off — with consequences.

And there's one more element to the physical demands of time and stress: not losing play and rest time. We all need to play and rest. Everyone needs to set aside some time each week to just go and do what it is they like best to do. To stop all playtime is to become vulnerable to fatigue, burnout, and illness.

Managing the mental drain of focusing so hard on our parents' needs is the second challenge. And that drain is real, even if we don't notice it. It's an unwelcome but constant companion. It eats at us and affects our ability for sound judgment and expected behaviour. A tired, cluttered brain isn't one that's going to make sound, logical decisions. It is one, however, that'll lead us into trouble faster than almost anything else.

For example, I know that I'm not as tolerant right now as I should be — with almost anyone. That bothers me, and I tell myself that I've got to watch it, but it's hard. I find I'm talking too much to too many people about what I'm experiencing. On one hand, it's probably therapeutic for me; on the other hand, I can imagine that in some cases I'm wearing out my welcome. People have their own problems and challenges to face, and clients have their own needs. So by dousing them with a stream of my personal woe, I'm not doing them any favours.

The key, it seems to me, is to understand and acknowledge the mental drain that comes with more involved caregiving, especially when a parent is suffering from physical or emotional problems. When the mental drain level soars, it's critical to take a break somehow, in some way — perhaps a quiet day, a short trip, or some kind of change to give the head and heart a break from the tension and pressure.

The third challenge — managing the frustration and guilt we feel as matters worsen — is a tough one. Feeling frustration and guilt is a natural part of caring for and loving our parents. But when either or both is physically or mentally ill, there's only so much we can do, and it's important to recognize and come to terms with that fact. While we can be supportive, while we can spend a lot of time and energy to help them, we can't turn back the clock and we can't fix the unfixable. We can be responsive and responsible, but we can't blame ourselves for what isn't our doing.

I know I'm battling frustration and guilt right now. I'm busy second-guessing what I should have done in the past couple of years and brooding over what else I could be doing right now. But when I look at it dispassionately, there really isn't much. I give, on all levels, as much as I can, and I have to accept that there's no more I can give, short of giving up my life and focusing totally on theirs. And that's not what a parent-child relationship is all about. Rather, I keep reminding myself, that relationship is supposed to be about our parents helping to rear and nurture us to a point where we launch into our own world, to seek our own course.

That's why all of us who strive to help our parents must acknowledge that we will do the best we can, but we will not suffer guilt trips. I'm learning this the hard way because my mother is trying to induce guilt right now. Demented or not, Alzheimer's or not, she's really working me over. For a long time, I didn't understand or recognize that. Now I do. That doesn't mean I love her any less; it only means I'm finally getting smarter and learning how to deal with it better.

As I near my destination, I conclude that the three challenges we face are real and threats to all of us. I've learned so much, the hard way, over the past few months. I know I've got to manage as best I can, and with the help of Gail and my children and our ever-expanding number of medical and social worker specialists, I will. But I do have to be self-ish to the extent that I manage my priorities and give myself permission to look after me.

It's as simple and as complex as that.

August 1, 2001

Today is my mother's birthday. She's eighty-seven.

This morning, Gail and I drive into the city, she, for appointments, and me, to take my mother to her noon appointment with the psychi-atric doctor. I arrive a few minutes early to pick her up and find her tense and apprehensive. I assure her all will be right, and she snaps back that this is her birthday. My father tells me he's tired, and my mother complains that no one's called to wish her a happy birthday. I remind her that their friends know not to call before early afternoon, but this doesn't wash with her. She's clearly miffed that her birthday isn't being celebrated as she thinks it should be.

We pack up my mother and her walker and I take her back to the hospital, arriving at the geriatric psychiatry wing right on time. On the way I had to listen to my mother tell me how I was late to pick her up, and how Gail says I'm always late for everything, and how it seems I can't manage my time very well, and more. After waiting a while, the doctor arrives again in a breeze of energy, does a few things, and again asks me to come to the same office to talk about how my mother coped over the past twenty-four hours. I tell him I'm not sure, since I wasn't there, and I call my father to ask. He tells me in Hungarian, and I tell the doctor in English, that she was pretty tired and calm, and all things con-sidered, everything worked out rather well.

After my report, he asks me to get my mother, which I do. He then asks her how she feels and a lot of other questions that, as I listen, make it clear he's probing to determine how mentally lucid she is. He explains again to her what medication to take and gives her a list and a prescrip-tion for one new pill (to help her relax more and sleep better). He says he's arranged for a nurse to see my mother twice a week and that he wants me to make an appointment for her to see a geriatric psychiatrist next week. Finally, he says he's signing a discharge order and that my mother is free to go.

My mother is reasonably calm through the meeting, saying that she understands everything and is delighted to do everything. We all smile a lot and shake hands, and my mother and I head back down the long hall to the security door. And as we walk down the hall, she pushing her walker and me walking next to her, she tells me again how all that's happened has been a set-up — a conspiracy — organized to do something I don't quite understand.

Once I get her back into the car, we stop at the pharmacy to drop off the prescription, and I tell her we'll have a birthday lunch. She says that would be nice and that she'd like a bowl of hot soup, but she doesn't want to go anywhere that anyone will recognize her because she can't handle the shame. I ignore this and take her to a nice suburban mall restaurant she knows. We study the menu, and my mother says she doesn't want any soup. We study the menu some more, and she says she doesn't want any kind of chicken dish, of which there are a lot. I suggest a spinach salad, and she agrees. We order and talk and it's nice and comfortable.

I tell her stories about our friends, and she asks a lot of questions.

Lunch arrives, and my mother digs in and eats like she hasn't seen food in a long time. Bits and pieces stick to her chin and some falls in her lap, but I say nothing.

We have a very nice time, and I'm thankful and pleased. Then, I lead her to a bench in one of the mall hallways and ask her to wait while I charge off to buy a few grocery items they need. When I get back, laden with bags, she's agitated. She needs toothpaste, she tells me — toothpaste she's asked me to get but I haven't. So I rush off to do that. When I get back, she tells me that she's tired and wants to go home because my father must surely be missing her and needing her attention. After all, my mother tells me, he's so fragile and wonderful, but she does wish he'd stop behaving so badly.

It's very hot out. We load into the car, crank up the air conditioning, and set off. We stop to pick up her new prescription and then drive to my parents' house. When we get inside, all hell breaks loose. She's suddenly very agitated and abusive. Everything is wrong. No one cares about her. It's her birthday and no one's called. She's ashamed to talk to anyone because she's been in a place that's locked up and her friends all know that. Where is the surprise party I said I'd arranged? And so on it goes. Then she tries on her birthday present — a new sweatsuit — and it doesn't fit right, and that sets her off some more. My mother tells me with quite some intensity that she's got a lot of clothes, but none that fit right, and all are old and worn. She sternly scolds their helper for holding her arm as she walks, telling her that she'll call for help when she needs it.

My father looks wan again. Sitting in the living room, he tells me how tired he is and that he's taken some Aspirin because he can feel pressure on his heart.

I just want out of there. It gets worse when my mother asks why I'm holding a container of her pills. I tell her it's one that's been replaced by what we just picked up and that we should throw it away, but she wants to study it and hold it as "evidence." I make the serious mistake of pulling it out of her hands and tossing it into the wastepaper basket. This leads to a major confrontation with her saying she doesn't need her pills anyway, how her diabetes has been cured, and that no one is calling to wish her a happy birthday.

I backtrack, but it's not enough, and so I improvise as best I can. But the damage is done, and I did it, and so I tell her I'm going downtown to pick up Gail and her other birthday surprises, and we'll be back.

Two hours later my father answers the door, looking even paler than he was earlier in the day. He says my mother is in her bedroom. Gail and I go to see her and Gail wishes my mother a happy birthday. My mother says she's tired and wants to rest and tells us to go away. Gail shows her the flower arrangement she brought and the cake with my mother's name inscribed. My mother wants to know why Gail didn't call her during the past week. And so we go again in a futile circle of senseless and unsatisfying conversation.

Gail tells my mother she'll put the flowers in a vase, and she leaves the room while I sit by her and talk nicely about our day. My mother, though, is focused on my father — how he's being so mean to her while she's being so forgiving. We talk about this for a few minutes, and my mother says that what she needs is to hear my father say that he loves her and that he's sorry about what he's done. Of course, he's said this a number of times over the past days, but she needs to hear it again, so I go to my father, who's sitting in the living room, and explain that he has to do it again. He's tired and wants to rest, but he props himself up, shuffles down the hall to her bedroom, and says it all one more time. I ask her to stand and for them to hug and kiss, which they do. And then my mother starts again about how my father refuses to confess his bad behaviour. As I look at him, I feel a pang in my heart because I can see the hurt and the weariness on his face.

We all head back to the living room where Gail's sitting. For the next half-hour, we try to make pleasant conversation about nothing in particular and admire the flower arrangement. My mother keeps delving into the most recent black hole in her mind, but she seems to be more subdued. Finally, Gail and I hug and kiss my mother and father and leave.

In the car, I call a couple of my parents' friends who understand my mother's condition. I remind them it's her birthday and ask them to call her.

And that's the way the day closes.

Tonight, as I write this, I dread the thought of the phone ringing. I don't want to hear any news. I'm tired. I'm dejected. I'm worried. I'm lost. I don't know what comes next, but whatever it is, I fear it.

On that note that I'm going to head off to sleep, convinced that tomorrow another chapter will unfold in the drama of our lives — a chapter that, if we're all fortunate, will be calmer, but who knows for sure?

SEPTEMBER 11, 2001

Today I took my mother to the geriatric psychiatrist who's now seeing her for the second time since I brought her home from the hospital six weeks ago. They have a wonderful visit. My mother seems at ease and sharp as a tack.

My mother talks about her memory — how she'd like to improve her ability to remember especially near-term events and issues. The doctor then asks if she'd mind taking the same test she's taken four times in the past two years that measures her cognitive abilities. My mother agrees.

The results genuinely surprise the doctor. Two years ago, on a scale that tops at thirty points, she scored about twenty-four. The next time she scored twenty-two, the third time she slipped to eighteen, and on the fourth test, some six months later, she was at a dangerous fourteen. The lower the number, the greater the short-term memory loss, and at fourteen, she was in serious trouble of having little retention and much confusion. And today her score is twenty-five — an amazing turnaround.

In fact, the doctor tells my mother that there's no need for him to see her for two months now, because he feels she's so much better and that her mind seems so much sharper. This is good news all around.

On the drive home, I tell my mother how proud I am of her and her progress. I explain that all the trauma of the past months is regrettable: having to take her to the hospital, having her tested, and living through all the personal emotional turmoil we all experienced. She tells me that she understands and that she knows she's for the moment better, both physically and emotionally.

I have dinner with my parents and go for a short walk with my father, who next week marks his ninety-sixth birthday. And then I head home with the fervent hope that we've stabilized and that, God willing, things can be calm and all right for a time.

Yet there's always the nagging reality that both my mother and father are old and at risk, and we just don't know what tomorrow will bring.

MAY 2, 2004

My father died during the night. Alone. At home, in his bedroom. At peace with himself, I fervently hope.

But let me backtrack.

It's been now nearly three years since we started writing the first edition of this book, and at the time I was living in fear and confusion because of my mother's condition and eventual forced hospitalization.

My mother did improve for a while. For nearly a year, she was reasonably well. And then she started a steep downward slide again.

By early fall 2002, she was totally immobile. We rented a Hoyer Lift to get her in and out of bed and used a travel wheelchair to move her around in the house. My mother seemed to decline by the day, to the point where her words were intelligible, she was totally incontinent, and she had to be spoon-fed by my parents' caregivers.

It was painful to watch, and we were again into a new crisis.

She demanded to sleep with my father but would wake him at all hours, to talk or in no uncertain terms to demand that they get dressed to go somewhere — catch a train, escape, or whatever strange thought crossed her troubled mind.

Their family physician had decided to leave his practice some months before, and we had a new family physician in place: Dr. Gregory Gelman, a young man who had started his practice just a year earlier. From the first visit onward, he was as patient and caring as the day is long. He always made time for my parents when I took them for appointments. But he also was concerned about my mother.

He recommended yet another assessment for my mother by our local geriatric assessment team. He booked examinations. And given all the results — which indicated my mother may be suffering from the Alzheimer's disease — he finally urged that we get her into a facility where a sound, longer-term assessment and observation could be conducted.

So we got her on a wait-list for the neurological unit at Baycrest Hospital. After some weeks of waiting, the call came: get her in the next day and expect her to stay for at least a few weeks.

This time my mother didn't resist. We arranged for an ambulance, which was to arrive at eight o'clock, and it finally got there at eleven o'clock. I was at Baycrest, waiting at the unit for her arrival.

She was confused and afraid: that was obvious.

And from mid-September through late December, my mother was a resident at Baycrest's amazing neurological unit. Week by week, there was a steady improvement in my mother's overall condition. At least once a week, I took my father to visit her for an hour or two. I arranged for some of her friends to see her from time to time and for her to get her hair done weekly. I visited most every day, wheeling her around, talking with her, just being there for her as best I could. Gail went to see her as often as she could, too.

Eventually, she was walking again, with the aid of a walker and loads of physiotherapy. She was feeding herself. She was no longer as incontinent. Her speech was much more normal. In short, she was in remarkably better shape than she had been in when she entered Baycrest.

Meanwhile, my father continued living at home, in reasonably good health, with around-the-clock support. But he was depressed. That was obvious. His failing eyesight troubled him hugely, and my mother's hospitalization was a hurtful forced separation that gnawed at him. It was like he felt guilty about being in the comfort of his home while my mother was hospitalized.

Just before Christmas, she was released on the condition that if things didn't work out well at home she would be readmitted. But things did work out reasonably well. For a few months. Part of the condition of her being at home was that she get up at a regular time, take her medications at given times, and be active; that she join a seniors' centre for regular activities; and that she exercise daily.

However, by early spring my mother refused to get up until at least early afternoon, often refused to take her medications on time, and definitely refused to go to any seniors' centre, let alone exercise. My mother began haranguing my father again, moving into his bed and staying there, often not wanting to get up at all. She wouldn't let my father sleep at night, and even during the day she would wake him from a nap to talk. And she kept pointing out that this was her house, her domain, and that all others had to follow her wishes.

She was, more often then not, agitated and verbally combative.

My father clearly was suffering from the stress and stain of it all. He finally asked me do something to relieve the tension he was feeling. Although it was obviously a huge moral dilemma for him, by April my father asked me to see if we could get my mother back into Baycrest. It took a while, but we got my mother readmitted to Baycrest on May 9, 2003.

And the whole cycle started again. The visits: me often, Gail as often as possible, my father at least weekly. The treatments. The jiggling and juggling of medications. New CT scans. And while my mother responded somewhat, it was not the same as before. There was progress and improvement yet again, but not to the same extent as the first time.

The long and short of it was that the medical team recommended that for her own good and safety my mother should not return home again, that she should be placed in a nursing home.

More conversations with my father. He understood intellectually, but it obviously troubled him emotionally. Me, too. It's the one place they both said they never wanted to be.

I then began a torrid round of reconnaissance visits to nursing homes that were in reasonable proximity to my parents' house. Most of what I saw, I didn't like. Some places were just too big, too impersonal. Some places looked nice, bright and new, but there was a "feeling" missing from the staff: to me, they were just putting in time, and the connection with residents was limited to the least that had to be done. Some places smelled of urine, and I was startled to the core by the dozens of elderly people I saw with heads lolling, strapped into wheel-chairs, just existing — no, barely subsisting, with little dignity and even less perceived respect.

If I had to have my mother in a nursing home, I wanted it to be a good one.

And I finally found one, recommended by the Community Care Access Centre liaison person who works out of Baycrest. She said there might be an opening at a place called Thompson House, actually very near my parents' house. She gave me a name and a number, and I called and hurried to visit.

Thompson House is a small facility, home to a hundred and change elderly people who live on three levels, reflecting the need for relatively independent living, assisted living, and full-care living. My mother was a full-care candidate.

I got the tour — yet another one. But this place felt good, smelled good. The staff seemed to be caring. They knew the names of all who lived there and had a good word, a smile, a pat, and patience for all. By now, I knew what to look for, and I found it at Thompson House.

I rushed to tell my father. He wasn't happy about it, but he con-curred this might be best.

So, on July 16, 2003, my mother was moved to Thompson House, her new and, most likely, final home.

My mother chose to dislike the place from the start. Yet today she's in better shape (except for her weight) than she has been since our odyssey to find the best care for her began three years ago. The place has lived up to all our expectations. The staff is genuine: the caring, the attention, the ambiance are real. Yes, it's small and tight for space. Yes, she has to share a room. Yes, there is too much TV time. Yes, it's not like home. But my mother looks better, does better, and *is* better than she has been in years as she approaches her ninetieth birthday.

Her condition seems stable, and with her new medication, her near-term memory is much better. Friends visit her. And she's made a few new friends at Thompson House.

But her complaints never cease. I know I have to listen to them, deal with them, accept them as part and parcel of what is and isn't right in her mind. And in her mind she is just fine, only all the others who are there are in some way mentally or physically unwell. And each resident on the fourth floor seems to think that's precisely the case with all their fellow residents.

From her move to Thompson House through to Christmas, I took my father at least once a week to see my mother.

But by November he was frailer, more agitated, and more restless. I took him for another visit to his geriatric psychiatrist, who prescribed a new antidepressant medication. The medication seemed to work at first, but the agitation and depression kept building. In early December the psychiatrist said we should increase the dosage, which we did, with no positive results.

By early January, my father seemed to be in worse shape. His caregiver was worried about him, as were we. But we were assured the medication would help and advised to give him yet more tablets at night.

Then, in early March, he just didn't want to get out of bed one morning.

And that was the beginning of the end.

I talked with Dr. Gelman, who made a house call to see him. He had tests conducted. The results: his system was strong, but he had a bladder infection.

Meanwhile, my daughter, Andrea, who is a marketing representative for a pharmaceutical company, started to worry about her grandfather and did an in-depth search of the antidepressant medication he was given. Her conclusion: the higher dosage we were told was acceptable to give him actually conflicted with his Parkinson's disease. I called our pharmacist, who checked with a pharmacological database and concurred that the dosage was way too high.

I checked with Dr. Gelman. He agreed, and immediately put him on another drug. I called and emailed the information to the geriatric psychiatrist, left another message some months ago, and to this day I have never heard back from him.

So whether it was the medication, the bladder infection — which in the elderly can cause numerous unwanted side effects, such as delusion — his decision that his life had lasted long enough, or whatever combination of these factors, my father started on his personal journey to death.

He ate less and less. He rejected all help. He remained in bed, sometimes quite lucid, and more often in some faraway place only he understood. He was on a daily sodium chloride drip and had a condom catheter attached to him.

Dr. Gelman came to see him weekly. He and I spoke numerous times about the options: to be aggressive (read hospitalization), or passive (read keep him at home and make him as comfortable as possible). I opted for keeping my father at home. In his lucid periods, when I asked, my father said he wanted to stay at home. I agreed with him. There was nothing they could've done in a hospital to make him better; he wouldn't walk again, let alone dance again, or think any better again, or do much of anything again.

Dr. Gelman and I also discussed the option of tube feeding. Aside from the discomfort of the process, I had real trouble grasping what benefit that might offer, other than making him live longer than he might wish. Keeping him alive would have been mainly for my benefit, not for his; to tube feed him really would've been an act of selfishness on my part.

Tube feeding begs the debate of the sanctity of life versus the quality of life, given any significant recovery was highly unlikely.

As he faded more and more, I shared memories from my childhood and fun and meaningful experiences together, in the hope of giving him some pleasurable mental moments and a sense of satisfaction. I often rubbed his neck and back and massaged his feet and legs, which he enjoyed greatly.

In my heart, I so wanted him to be better, but in my head I knew he wouldn't be.

I reported on his condition to my mother on my regular visits. My mother clearly had mixed emotions, but as often as not she was remarkably astute given her condition. She observed that her husband was old, that he had lived a long life, and that he should not suffer.

A few weeks before his death, I arranged for my mother to have a visit home so they could share some time together. The next visit was scheduled for today. I cancelled the visit when I knew my father had died. There was no sense in my mother seeing him dead.

Watching him wilt away, listening to him ramble on about people and events from his distant past or some terrible event imagined in his mind, and feeling him ever so slowly but surely sliding toward the personal conclusion of his life was an agonizing experience for me.

And I knew I must accept that he would die in the near future.

My profound hope was that he would die at peace with himself, in the knowledge that he did so many wonderful things, and that he was respected and loved by those of us near to him.

And I hoped I would have the strength and resolve to grieve as I must, celebrate all we shared, carry good memories, and march on. Because that's the way of the real world, like it or not.

So now my father is dead. He hasn't "left us" or "moved to the beyond" or "passed on" or anything like that. He is simply dead, and if there is an afterlife, his soul is bound to be there, and I guess and hope he'll know how much he meant to me and always will. And I look at his ashen face and kiss his cold forehead, and I cry. Because crying is good when the pain is deep. I am alone with his body in his bedroom, and this is a safe and sure place full of flooding memories.

I think about how Gail and I will tell my mother, because Gail said she wants to be there, to support both of us.

I am waiting for the people from the funeral home to take away the stiffened corpse of a frail old man whom I loved and love even at this moment, just as I love my children and Gail and my mother.

I sit alone in the kitchen of my parents' house, and tears dribble down my face.

A huge slice of my life is gone forever.

May 8, 2004

Today, we held a memorial service for my father.

I picked up the urn with his ashes just hours ago from the funeral home. It felt totally weird carrying my father's burned remains in an urn, in a velvet bag.

We had a memorable service at E.P. Taylor Place, adjacent to Thompson House, so my mother could be there. Nearly thirty of my parents' aging friends were in attendance, and our Hungarian Presbyterian minister delivered a moving eulogy that was meaningful and heartfelt.

My mother handled the event better than I did. Sitting next to her, I stroked her arm, and she seemed to be all right.

On my other side, my daughter, Andrea, and I held hands through the eulogy.

And I thought about my other two children and wished that they could have been there, because my father so much loved them, too.

And then we had finger foods and cheese and fruit and talked and shared memories and felt so vulnerable without ever expressing it, because we are the next wave of the aging and elderly who will one by one die.

August 1, 2004

Today is my mother's ninetieth birthday.

Gail, close family friend Klari, and I organized a surprise birthday party for her, in the same room where just three months ago we held the memorial service for my father.

Twelve aging friends of my mother, my daughter, Andrea, her husband, Julian, and Gail and I were there to fete her. One friend who so wanted to be there had been diagnosed with terminal cancer just two weeks ago and is now in palliative care.

It was a good event, a wonderful event. My mother smiled a lot, looked charming and not at all her age, and was at times totally "there" and sometimes totally confused.

Such is her life now — slipping into her personal worlds, where sometimes she is amazed about things I tell her that she just doesn't remember, and sometimes sweet and patient, and sometimes irritated and combative.

I just never know how she'll be on any given day.

But my mother always looks longingly at the large photo taken by Gail some five years ago that I mounted near her bed, depicting my parents leaning on each other for support and smiling and looking like a lovely aging couple. And so often she tells me that she's reminded by that photo just how much she loved my father, and how old she now is, and how much our little family means to her.

When she says that, I can feel the tears welling up, and I love my parents all the more, carrying the hurt of my father's death and filled with hope that my mother will be as well as possible, for as long as possible.

And I guess that's what parents are all about. All about this history we carry with us, from birth to our own death, even if the images fade and the memories wane.

LESSONS LEARNED

Friend, colleague, and co-author with me of another book, Dr. Harvey Silver always talks about the difference between tender loving care and tough loving care. An organizational psychologist, Harvey likes to explain that tender loving care is easy: we just give what's wanted, do what's expected, and keep opting out of the difficult decisions that make us all accountable and leaders in the truest sense. On the other hand, tough loving care demands making hard decisions that take us out of our zones of comfort. Tough loving care means that while we respect a person, we don't accept problem behaviours and attitudes.

When I apply those concepts to my own experience with my parents — and in particular to my mother's problems — I think the biggest, most valuable lesson I learned is that we must abide by our parents' wishes, but only so long as they don't harm themselves or each other or anyone else. There comes a critical point in time when we have to take control and do the undoable: when we have to bite the bullet and make decisions that hurt but, in fact, will help. Had I not taken the painful step of having my mother hospitalized against her wishes, we may well have had a family crisis that could have cost us more emotionally than we could manage. Had I not agreed that my mother is best off in a nursing home, I think she would be in much worse condition today than she is. And had I not listened to my father's wishes about wanting to remain at home during his final days, I think I would have done him a disservice and made those days much more trying and painful.

I have also learned that tolerance is golden. In the case of my mother, I needed to accept her concerns and fears. I didn't do that very well for too long, and as a result I probably caused more mutual pain than was necessary. But I don't think I understood that as well at the outset of her difficulties as I do today.

It's a delicate balancing act to exercise tough loving care. It's knowing when to intervene and where to draw the line. Common sense should've told me that, but in retrospect I see there just wasn't much common sense evident when the emotions of the moment tended to overwhelm good reasoning.

Another lesson I learned is the need to better understand what the doctors are and aren't saying. They're trying to do the best they can, and I was touched by the genuine concern and eagerness of most to find the best possible ways to help my mother and my father. But because they have their own pressures, and because many well-intentioned doctors can't seem to explain things in a patient, clear way, too often we don't understand what we hear. I learned to keep asking, to seek further clarification, to, as they say, drill down. I think I became somewhat of a pest with my persistent questioning, yet it was only because I kept asking questions that I got a much better picture of what we were facing.

I also learned to slow down with my parents and to try to talk more slowly and more clearly. The more intense I was, the more agitated they'd become, and we'd end up in confrontational situations. While what I was saying at any time to my parents was clear to me, I was operating in my paradigm, not theirs, which I found frustrating, but which for too long I didn't understand. So the more calmly I spoke, the more receptive they became. It's such a simple lesson, but one that I've learned the hard way.

A rather bitter and belated lesson struck home much more recently. And that is to be much more careful about the caregivers one engages. For several years, we had a procession of people in and out of my parents' home, some from agencies and others we recruited. I never thought too much about it, but I discovered during the process of cleaning out their home and moving everything that a number of valuable items were missing. Most painful was the realization that my mother's diamond ring, worth quite a bit of money, was gone. I don't know how to guard against such situations, let alone prevent them. The fact is that when there are so many caregivers involved over a longer period of time, chances are there will be one who walks away with something.

With my father's death, I discovered that I was no longer seized with fear when any of our phones rang. For several years now, starting with my mother's initial outburst, I've lived in constant concern every time the home, office, or especially my cell phone rang. I just never knew who would be calling, but always automatically assumed it was the caregiver, the nurse, a doctor, or someone who was about to tell me something I didn't want to hear or know.

Now, I feel less trepidation when the phones ring. I'm more eager to answer, knowing my mother is safe and relatively well, and that she is the only parent I now need to be concerned about.

And I've learned that there is only so much I can do for my parents. I can help make them safe and comfortable. I can ensure their financial matters are in order. I can be there for them, as often as I can. But I can't live their lives or abdicate my life for them. I may want to, but it won't work, and it won't help.

Guilt plays such a large part in the process of caring for our parents. I know now that guilt only dissipates my energy and abilities. Yet guilt about whether or not I'm doing or have done the best I can for too long dominated me. So perhaps the most important lesson of all that I've learned is to manage my sense of guilt and not let it overwhelm me. If I can honestly say that I am doing the best I can for my parents, while maintaining some good measure of a personal and professional life, then I should not feel guilty at all. Because I'm helping make my parents' lives as full and rich and good as possible. And that meets their expectations (whether they acknowledge it or not) and fulfills my sense of love and responsibility.

PERSONAL PARENTING PLANNER

WHY A PERSONAL PARENTING PLANNER?

Inevitably, there will come a time when you'll have to act promptly to help your parents in some type of emergency or a family crisis. When that time comes, you'll want to know how to access people and documents to best support your parents' needs at that moment. If you have to start searching for — or guessing about — the information that's needed, you'll lose valuable time and only fuel your own level of anxiety and tension.

That's why we've developed and included this Personal Parenting Planner. At first glance, filling in all the blanks in this extensive planning tool may seem a daunting task. Or, for some, it may appear to be an unnecessary, or even frivolous, time-consuming task. But we want to assure you that the Personal Parenting Planner will be an invaluable tool and resource for you at some point, in some way.

Consider all the corporations, hospitals, government departments, and most other organizations that have complex, comprehensive crisis management plans. The plans that are good all have a lot of lists — where to find people, important information about the organization, needed resources, and more. Those plans and lists exist because experience has shown that when there's any emergency situation or a full-blown crisis, it's critical to be able to find the accurate information needed to make decisions — and to find it quickly. Time becomes an essential factor, and when there is a crisis — as there will be at some point in the future — most of us won't know or remember half of what we need to have in hand.

So whether on the macro level of large organizations or the micro level of a family, having the information you need, a good situation analysis, and a course of action to follow can make the difference between doing the right things the right way and trying to wing it and most likely making matters worse.

Case in point: shortly after the first edition of *Parenting Your Parents* was published, a woman in Victoria bought a copy of the book and discovered this section. Her mother had died a couple of years ago, and she decided to do some planning with her father, who was at first reluctant but finally agreed. They'd worked their way through most of this planner when he suffered a major stroke that left him totally incapacitated. The woman reported that had she not gathered the information she did, she wouldn't have known where her father's house keys were, or where he banked, or about his pension plans.

Now, it's your turn.

There are two parts to the Personal Parenting Planner. Part 1 is an inventory — a fact-gathering mission to collect useful information you'll need at some point and to assess family capabilities, challenges, and commitment. Some of the considerations you'll be asked to tackle may be uncomfortable; however, now is the time to address them. And to best help your parents and yourself, please be candid and honest; it's the only way this assessment will help you in your decision-making. Remember that no one else will see what you mark unless you elect to share it. Part 2 is an action plan of what you'll do now and later — for your parents, and for yourself.

In Section 3 (Taking Inventory) of Part 1, we've added a scoring process to twenty of the statements regarding both your mother and father, ranging from six (in good shape) to zero (you don't know). As you work your way through this section, please circle the appropriate number opposite the statement you're being asked to judge. You'll note that in some cases the same numerical value is given to more than one option in response to completing a statement, and in some cases the numbers are not in sequential order. This is intentional; some options merit the same value because of the implications, and some statements offer options that are more severe in their implications.

When you've added up your numbers, please return to this page to find out what your score means in general terms, recognizing that this is a relatively subjective assessment that nevertheless will offer a good guideline.

Scoring

If your total is between 120 and 72 points for either parent: Things right now seem to be fairly stable and sound. This is an excellent time to talk with your parents to plan for the future and to come to understand their wishes.

If your total is between 71 and 41 points for either parent: There's a definite trend toward changes happening; your parent is more vulnerable. Now is the time to take a closer look at his or her capabilities and needs, and in the very near future to determine what kind of added assistance will be needed.

If your total is 40 points or under for either parent: Your parent needs immediate added support and help. Please act promptly and decisively, getting all the sound advice and support you need.

Note: If you scored more than seven zeros for either parent, then you aren't in touch with him or her. You must evaluate your level of involvement and your willingness to be much more supportive.

We've tried to make the Personal Parenting Planner as comprehensive and broad-based as possible, but remember: the planner will be helpful and relevant only if it's updated as information changes. Don't just file it in your desk once you've completed it. Be sure to remember to mark down changes as they occur, and make a note on your calendar to review it every few months.

TAKING INVENTORY

Last updated on: _____

SECTION 1: MY PARENTS' ADVISORS AND FRIENDS

In this section, list full names, addresses, telephone/cell and fax numbers, and email addresses of those people who help or advise your parents or are good friends. If you don't have the information, now is the time to collect it!

Their family physician:

_____

_____

_____

Their health-related specialists:

_____

_____

_____

_____

Their clergy:

_____

_____

_____

Their lawyer:

_____

_____

_____

Their accountant:

_____

_____

_____

Their financial planner:

_____

_____

_____

Their life insurance agent:

_____

_____

_____

Their general insurance broker (_house, car, property_):

_____

_____

_____

Their bank:

_____

_____

_____

Types of accounts and account numbers:

_____

_____

_____

_____

_____

Safety deposit boxes (*location and number; location of keys*):

_____

_____

_____

Location of up-to-date wills:

_____

_____

_____

Location of living wills:

_____

_____

_____

Location of signed power of attorney documents:

_____

_____

_____

Their closest relatives:

_____

_____

_____

_____

_____

_____

_____

Their closest friends:

_____
_____
_____

Their immediate neighbours:

_____
_____
_____

They have made funeral arrangements through:

_____
_____
_____

They have made burial decisions, which are kept:

_____
_____
_____

Location of important family documents (including passports):

_____
_____
_____

SECTION 2: MY PARENT'S HEALTH CARE PLANS AND INCOME SOURCES

In this section, record the very important data about your parents' health coverage, life insurance particulars, and income sources. In case of illness or death, you'll need these to notify various agencies and companies about possible changes in benefit payments and reporting requirements.

Father's social insurance number: _____

Father's health card number: _____

Mother's social insurance number: _____

Mother's health card number: _____

Pension plan details:

_____

_____

_____

RRSP (Registered Retirement Savings Plan) details:

_____

_____

_____

CPP/QPP (Canada Pension Plan/Quebec Pension Plan) details:

_____

_____

_____

Guaranteed Income Supplement:

_____

_____

_____

Goods and Services Tax/Harmonized Sales Tax Credit (as allowable):

_____

_____

_____

Annuity plans:

_____

_____

_____

Optional health care coverage plans:

_____

_____

_____

Life insurance policies:

_____

_____

_____

SECTION 3: PROFILE OF MY PARENTS

This section is an inventory of the state of your parents' health, mindset, and observed behaviour right now. This can be a difficult section to complete. You must be objective and honest and make the best possible assumptions in some cases. The end result is a profile of each of your parents that will help you to better assess their current condition and allow you to better anticipate their personal mental and physical health needs in the immediate future.

Father

My father is ____ years old.

His health right now is:

☐	good	6
☐	stable	5
☐	questionable	4
☐	eroding	3
☐	not good	2
☐	poor	1
☐	don't know, but need to find out	0

His main health problems are:

_____

_____

_____

_____

_____

☐ don't know, but need to find out

To the best of my knowledge, his doctor thinks that my father is:

☐ doing well for his age		6
☐ has some minor problems		5
☐ has at least one major problem		3
☐ has very serious problems		1
☐ don't know, but need to find out		0

Mentally, my father is:

☐ sound		6
☐ gets confused now and then		4
☐ gets confused often		2
☐ fragile		1
☐ don't know, but need to find out		0

Physically, my father's ability to move is:

☐ independent and mobile		6
☐ relatively stable		5
☐ stable but at times unsure		5
☐ safer with a cane		4
☐ safer with a walker		3
☐ restricted to the use of a walker		2
☐ very limited		1
☐ don't know, but need to find out		0

If he's taking medication on a regular basis, he:

☐ is consistent and reliable		6
☐ sometimes forgets		5
☐ often forgets		3

☐ must be given pre-packaged doses 2
☐ must be administered medications 1
☐ don't know, but need to find out 0

Socially, my father is:

☐ active 6
☐ moderately active 5
☐ a bit passive 4
☐ passive 2
☐ reclusive 1
☐ don't know, but need to find out 0

With my mother, he is:

☐ supportive 6
☐ fairly supportive 5
☐ moderately supportive 5
☐ not very supportive 4
☐ passive 3
☐ unsupportive 2
☐ hostile 1
☐ don't know, but need to find out 0

With my spouse, he is:

☐ very comfortable 6
☐ somewhat comfortable 5
☐ not very comfortable 4
☐ somewhat uncomfortable 3
☐ very uncomfortable 2
☐ hostile 1
☐ not really sure, but need to find out 0

With my children, he is:

☐ kind and caring 6
☐ very involved 6
☐ somewhat involved 4
☐ mostly uninvolved 2

☐ totally uninvolved 1

☐ not really sure, but need to find out 0

With other immediate family, he is:

☐ very comfortable 6

☐ somewhat comfortable 5

☐ not very comfortable 4

☐ somewhat uncomfortable 3

☐ very uncomfortable 2

☐ hostile 1

☐ don't know, but need to find out 0

My family would likely characterize my father as:

☐ nice to be with most of the time 6

☐ nice to be with for shorter periods of time 4

☐ tolerable to be with from time to time 2

☐ not very nice to be with any time 1

Why? _____

_____

_____

☐ not really sure, but need to find out 0

Usually in appearance, he is:

☐ well groomed 6

☐ not too well groomed 5

☐ sloppy 3

☐ dishevelled 1

☐ don't know, but need to find out 0

He enjoys:

☐ hobbies that keep him occupied, which are 6

_____

_____

_____

_____

☐ some hobbies that interest him, which are   6

_____

_____

☐ a hobby that engages him periodically, which is   4

_____

☐ no hobbies   1
☐ don't know, but need to find out   0

He has:

☐ a number of friends he meets/talks with on a regular basis   6
☐ a few friends he meets/talks with on a regular basis   5
☐ one friend he meets/talks with on a regular basis   4
☐ a few friends he meets/talks with only infrequently   3
☐ no friends he meets/talks with on a regular basis   1
☐ don't know, but need to find out   0

He:

☐ gets out frequently to do things   6
☐ gets out from time to time to do things   5
☐ doesn't get out much   4
☐ rarely gets out of the house   2
☐ doesn't go out at all   1
☐ don't know, but need to find out   0

He:

☐ drives a car all the time   6
☐ drives a car at least once a week   5
☐ drives a car once in a while   4
☐ doesn't drive   3
☐ don't know, but need to find out   0

When he drives, he:

☐ drives safely   6
☐ occasionally loses his way   4
☐ often loses his way   2

☐ drives unsafely   1

☐ don't know, but need to find out   0

He:

☐ has a will that is current   6

☐ has a will that was written or updated within the
past five years   4

☐ __ has a will that was written a number of years ago
and has not been changed   2

☐ does not have a will   0

☐ don't know, but need to find out   0

He:

☐ has a living will that is current   6

☐ has a living will that was written or updated
within the pastfive years   4

☐ has a living will that was written a number of
years ago and has not been changed   2

☐ does not have a living will   0

☐ don't know, but need to find out   0

He:

☐ has given me power of attorney   6

☐ has not given me power of attorney   2

☐ has given power of attorney to _____   6

☐ don't know, but need to find out   0

Score Total: _____

Overall, I think my father right now is:

in a physical condition that can be best summarized as

_____

in an emotional condition that can best be summarized as

_____

and so the most important things I have to watch for are

_____

_____

Mother

My mother is __ years old.

Her health right now is:

☐ good		6
☐ stable		5
☐ questionable		4
☐ eroding		3
☐ not good		2
☐ poor		1
☐ don't know, but need to find out		0

Her main health problems are:

_____

_____

_____

_____

☐ don't know, but need to find out

To the best of my knowledge, her doctor thinks that my mother is:

☐ doing well for her age		6
☐ has some minor problems		5
☐ has at least one major problem		3
☐ has very serious problems		1
☐ don't know, but need to find out		0

Mentally, my mother is:

☐ sound		6
☐ gets confused now and then		4
☐ gets confused often		2
☐ fragile		1
☐ don't know, but need to find out		0

Physically, my mother's ability to move is:

- [ ] independent and mobile — 6
- [ ] relatively stable — 5
- [ ] stable but at times unsure — 5
- [ ] safer with a cane — 4
- [ ] safer with a walker — 3
- [ ] restricted to the use of a walker — 2
- [ ] very limited — 1
- [ ] don't know, but need to find out — 0

If she's taking medication on a regular basis, she:

- [ ] is consistent and reliable — 6
- [ ] sometimes forgets — 5
- [ ] often forgets — 3
- [ ] must be given pre-packaged doses — 2
- [ ] must be administered medications — 1
- [ ] don't know, but need to find out — 0

Socially, my mother is:

- [ ] active — 6
- [ ] moderately active — 5
- [ ] a bit passive — 4
- [ ] passive — 2
- [ ] reclusive — 1
- [ ] don't know, but need to find out — 0

With my father, she is:

- [ ] supportive — 6
- [ ] fairly supportive — 5
- [ ] moderately supportive — 5
- [ ] not very supportive — 4
- [ ] passive — 3
- [ ] unsupportive — 2
- [ ] hostile — 1
- [ ] don't know, but need to find out — 0

With my spouse, she is:

☐ very comfortable		6
☐ somewhat comfortable		5
☐ not very comfortable		4
☐ somewhat uncomfortable		3
☐ very uncomfortable		2
☐ hostile		1
☐ not really sure, but need to find out		0

With my children, she is:

☐ kind and caring		6
☐ very involved		6
☐ somewhat involved		4
☐ mostly uninvolved		2
☐ totally uninvolved		1
☐ not really sure, but need to find out		0

With other immediate family, she is:

☐ very comfortable		6
☐ somewhat comfortable		5
☐ not very comfortable		4
☐ somewhat uncomfortable		3
☐ very uncomfortable		2
☐ hostile		1
☐ don't know, but need to find out		0

My family would likely characterize my mother as:

☐ nice to be with most of the time		6
☐ nice to be with for shorter periods of time		4
☐ tolerable to be with from time to time		2
☐ not very nice to be with any time		1

Why?_____

_____

_____

☐ not really sure, but need to find out		0

Usually in appearance, she is:

- ☐ well groomed — 6
- ☐ not too well groomed — 5
- ☐ sloppy — 3
- ☐ dishevelled — 1
- ☐ don't know, but need to find out — 0

She enjoys:

- ☐ hobbies that keep her occupied, which are — 6

_____

_____

_____

_____

- ☐ some hobbies that interest her, which are — 6

_____

_____

_____

- ☐ a hobby that engages her periodically, which is — 4

_____

- ☐ no hobbies — 1
- ☐ don't know, but need to find out — 0

She has:

- ☐ a number of friends she meets/talks with on a regular basis — 6
- ☐ a few friends she meets/talks with on a regular basis — 5
- ☐ one friend she meets/talks with on a regular basis — 4
- ☐ a few friends she meets/talks with only infrequently — 3
- ☐ no friends she meets/talks with on a regular basis — 1
- ☐ don't know, but need to find out — 0

She:

- ☐ gets out frequently to do things — 6
- ☐ gets out from time to time to do things — 5
- ☐ doesn't get out much — 4
- ☐ rarely gets out of the house — 2

☐ doesn't go out at all   1
☐ don't know, but need to find out   0

She:

☐ drives a car all the time   6
☐ drives a car at least once a week   5
☐ drives a car once in a while   4
☐ doesn't drive   3
☐ don't know, but need to find out   0

When she drives, she:

☐ drives safely   6
☐ occasionally loses his way   4
☐ often loses his way   2
☐ drives unsafely   1
☐ don't know, but need to find out   0

She:

☐ has a will that is current   6
☐ has a will that was written or updated within
the past five years   4
☐ has a will that was written a number of years ago
and has not been changed   2
☐ does not have a will   0
☐ don't know, but need to find out   0

She:

☐ has a living will that is current   6
☐ has a living will that was written or updated
within the past five years   4
☐ has a living will that was written a number of
years ago and has not been changed   2
☐ does not have a living will   0
☐ don't know, but need to find out   0

She:

☐ has given me power of attorney 6
☐ has not given me power of attorney 2
☐ has given power of attorney to _____ 6
☐ don't know, but need to find out 0

Score Total: _____

Overall, I think my mother right now is:

in a physical condition that can be best summarized as

_____

in an emotional condition that can best be summarized as

_____

and so the most important things I have to watch for are

_____

_____

My Parents Together

My parents are:

☐ married
☐ separated
☐ divorced

As a married couple they:

☐ get along well all of the time
☐ get along well most of the time
☐ have a fair amount of friction between them
☐ argue a lot
☐ argue all the time
☐ aren't very compatible
☐ don't know, but need to find out

As a separated or divorced couple they:

☐ have a relatively good relationship
☐ have a decent, respectful relationship

- ☐ have a relatively poor relationship
- ☐ don't have a relationship at all
- ☐ don't know, but need to find out

My parents:

- ☐ share most values and beliefs
- ☐ share some values and beliefs
- ☐ don't have as much in common as I thought
- ☐ are at odds over more than I'd assumed
- ☐ tolerate each other
- ☐ aren't close at all, when I think about it
- ☐ don't know, but need to find out

Financially, they are:

- ☐ very secure
- ☐ somewhat secure
- ☐ not very secure
- ☐ vulnerable
- ☐ don't know, but need to find out

They live in:

- ☐ a house
- ☐ an apartment
- ☐ a trailer home
- ☐ in a retirement home/community
- ☐ in an assisted living facility
- ☐ in a nursing home
- ☐ at our house
- ☐ at someone else's house (_____)

They get outside help from:

- ☐ a housekeeper (e.g., cleaning and cooking)
  - ☐ once a week
  - ☐ twice a week
  - ☐ three to five times a week
  - ☐ daily for several hours

☐ a homemaker (e.g., housekeeper duties plus care services such as dressing and bathing)
- ☐ once a week
- ☐ twice a week
- ☐ three to five times a week
- ☐ daily for several hours

☐ full-time in-home support

☐ live-in support

☐ don't know, but need to find out

In our family, the person they like the most is:

_____

In our family the person my father most trusts is:

_____

In our family, the person my mother most trusts is:

_____

Based on my analysis, it seems that my father's relationship with my mother can be described as being:

_____

_____

_____

Based on my analysis, it seems that my mother's relationship with my father can be described as being:

_____

_____

_____

Finally, based on my analysis, I think that the most important factors I have to consider, act on, or watch for are:

_____

_____

_____

SECTION 4: ME AND MY FAMILY

This section is an inventory of how prepared you and your siblings are. Because it's important to plan in advance, you're being asked to consider what challenges you may face, how you might help your parents, and how you might co-operate with your spouse and/or siblings to share responsibilities. Take time to think through your answers carefully. Keep in mind that defining clear goals and roles is just as vital in our personal lives as it is in business.

Me and My Spouse/Partner

I'm __ years old.

I'm:

- ☐ married
- ☐ living common-law
- ☐ living alone
- ☐ divorced and living alone
- ☐ in transition

My spouse/partner supports me in understanding my parents' needs and is willing to help:

- ☐ yes
- ☐ no
- ☐ not sure

If no, why not?

_____

_____

_____

_____

_____

If not sure, why not?

_____

_____

_____

What I need to do to enlist his/her support and help:

_____

_____

_____

My spouse/partner has his/her own parents to help, and so we must:

- ☐ define how we'll work together to provide care for both sets of parents
- ☐ define how much time we will allocate to each set of parents
- ☐ determine how we'll ensure we have time to spend with our children
- ☐ determine how we'll find time for ourselves
- ☐ agree on how to be mutually supportive in times of stress
- ☐ set aside some quiet time to talk this through and develop a mutually acceptable plan of action

My spouse/partner doesn't have his/her own parents to help, and so I can expect he/she will help me by:

- ☐ giving me moral support
- ☐ taking more time with the children to give me more time with my parents
- ☐ spending some time each week with my parents to give me time for other obligations
- ☐ assuming some activities (e.g., banking, etc.) to free up more of my time

My spouse/partner has his/her own children to help, and so we must:

- ☐ agree on how to manage all our relationships
- ☐ agree on how I can help with the children, and to what extent
- ☐ agree on how he/she can help with my parents, and to what extent
- ☐ ensure the children understand the new challenges we face

My Siblings

I have the following siblings:

- ☐ _____, who lives in _____, and when it comes to caring about our parent(s), feels that
_____.

- ☐ _____, who lives in _____, and when it comes to caring about our parent(s), feels that
_____.

- ☐ _____, who lives in _____, and when it comes to caring about our parent(s), feels that
_____.

- ☐ _____, who lives in _____, and when it comes to caring about our parent(s), feels that
_____.

(List other siblings as needed.)

_____

_____

_____

My siblings are committed to caring about my parent(s):

- ☐ absolutely
- ☐ firmly
- ☐ somewhat
- ☐ not very
- ☐ not at all

If there is a barrier/problem about caring for my parent(s), it's that:

- ☐ my parents don't want help, even though they need it
- ☐ we're not on especially good terms
- ☐ my work leaves me too little time for anything else
- ☐ my home life demands a lot of time and attention
- ☐ financially, we don't have extra money to spend on parental support of any kind
- ☐ I have a medical condition that will prevent me from providing a lot of hands-on support
- ☐ __ there is a lack of willingness among my siblings to help me
- ☐ other:

_____

_____

In terms of caring for my parents, that means:

_____

_____

_____

_____

_____

_____

My siblings and I have talked about what that implies in terms of time, energy, and resources:

- ☐ yes
- ☐ not very much
- ☐ not at all

We are clear and in agreement about what we will do with and for our parents:

- ☐ yes
- ☐ not very
- ☐ not at all

Fill in the following chart to evaluate your own and your siblings' ability to help your parent(s) with the tasks listed. Rank the tasks as 1=easy to do; 2=can do without much difficulty; 3=can't do very easily; 4=difficult to do; 5=impossible to do. You can use the filled-in chart to identify possible gaps in the care you and your siblings can provide to your parent(s).

TASK	ME	#1	#2	#3	#4
call regularly					
visit once a week					
visit more frequently					
take them to the bank					
take them for walks					
take them for drives					
take them to social events					
bring them to my house for a visit					
take them for doctors' appointments					
talk with their doctors					
drop off/pick up prescriptions					
grocery shop for them regularly					
take my them to hair appointments					
do repairs/maintenance around their house					
arrange home repairs					
cook for them once or twice a week					
prepare meals in advance for them weekly					

TASK	ME	#1	#2	#3	#4
help with paying bills					
help with financial matters					
help with tax returns					
arrange in-home support services					
monitor the quality of support services					
helping with garden and lawn care					
shovel snow					
other:_____					
other:_____					
other:_____					

The major challenge for me with helping my parent(s) is:

_____

_____

because:

_____

_____

_____

The major challenge for my sibling _____ with helping my parent(s) is:

_____

_____

because:

_____

_____

_____

The major challenge for my sibling _____ with helping my parent(s) is:

_____

_____

because:

_____

_____

_____

The major challenge for my sibling _____ with helping my parent(s) is:

_____

_____

because:

_____

_____

_____

The major challenge for my sibling _____ with helping my parent(s) is:

_____

_____

because:

_____

_____

_____

Given what I've discovered through this exercise, I can conclude that in the process of helping my parent(s), we will be able to do the following with consistency and care for as long as we're needed to support them:

_____

_____

_____

_____

_____

_____

_____

_____

Given what I've discovered through this exercise, I can conclude that in the process of helping my parent(s), we will not be able to do the following with consistency and care for whatever time we're needed to support them:

_____

_____

_____

_____

_____

_____

_____

_____

_____

As a result, we must think now about how to arrange for the following:

_____

_____

_____

_____

_____

_____

_____

_____

Finally, we have discussed and agree on who the lead sibling will be in the process of caring for our parents, recognizing and agreeing that the lead sibling will make daily decisions and consult with his/her siblings in dire circumstances but be responsible for the implementation of whatever actions must be taken. We have agreed that the lead sibling will be: _____.

PART 2

Action Plan

Last updated on: _____

SECTION 1: What I Need to Do or Plan for Right Now

Given what I know at the moment, MY FATHER needs in the near term: (*Rank the following as 1=highest priority; 2=important to implement soon; 3=must consider; 4=should address; 5=will probably need within the next 9-12 months.*)

- ☐ my/our added visibility and presence
- ☐ moral support
- ☐ help with day-to-day living
- ☐ a "time out" from his current environment to regain his mental and physical strength
- ☐ specialized medical attention
- ☐ in-home added support
- ☐ placement in an institution

Given what I know at the moment, MY MOTHER needs in the near term: (*Rank the following as 1=highest priority; 2=important to implement soon; 3=must consider; 4=should address; 5=will probably need within the next 9-12 months.*)

- ☐ my/our added visibility and presence
- ☐ moral support
- ☐ help with day-to-day living
- ☐ a "time out" from her current environment to regain her mental and physical strength
- ☐ specialized medical attention
- ☐ in-home added support
- ☐ placement in an institution

If one or both parents do not have an up-to-date will (within the past two years), I will:

- ☐ help one or both update a will
- ☐ arrange for a lawyer to see one or both to update a will
- ☐ encourage my parent(s) to update a will

If one or both parents do not have an up-to-date living will (within the past two years), I will:

- ☐ help one or both update living will
- ☐ arrange for a lawyer to see one or both to update a living will
- ☐ encourage my parent(s) to update a living will

If one or both parents do not have an up-to-date general and financial powers of attorney (within the past two years), I will:

- ☐ help one or both update their powers of attorney
- ☐ arrange for a lawyer to see one or both to update their powers of attorney
- ☐ encourage my parent(s) to update a their powers of attorney
- ☐ urge my parent(s) to arrange for such powers of attorney as soon as possible

We have discussed any special wishes my father may have regarding the kind and level of health care he expects, especially in defining how to handle the question of prolonging his life if he is in a critical condition.

- ☐ Yes, we have, and we have a clear understanding of his wishes.
- ☐ We've talked about it, but there is no clear direction.
- ☐ No, we haven't talked about it.

If not, I will _____

We have discussed any special wishes my mother may have regarding the kind and level of health care she expects, especially in defining how to handle the question of prolonging her life if she is in a critical condition.

- ☐ Yes, we have and have a clear understanding of his wishes.
- ☐ We've talked about it, but there is no clear direction.

☐ No, we haven't talked about it.
If not, I will _____

We have discussed funeral and burial wishes:

☐ yes
☐ no
If not, I will _____

We have discussed and prepared obituary notices:

☐ yes
☐ no
If not, I will _____

We have discussed how to distribute special mementoes, heirlooms, and other personal effects:

☐ yes
☐ no
If not, I will _____

SECTION 2: WHAT I WILL PROBABLY NEED TO DO IN THE NEAR FUTURE

Based on all I now know about my *father*, I believe that within the next two years, he will need the following (in order of priority):

1. _____
2. _____
3. _____
4. _____

Of these, I can provide the following:

1. _____
2. _____
3. _____
4. _____

Of these, I will need help with the following from other sources (see Resource Directory for support agencies):

Source: _____

Source: _____

Source: _____

Source: _____

Based on all I now know about my *mother*, I believe that within the next two years, she will need the following (in order of priority):

1. _____
2. _____
3. _____
4. _____

Of these, I can provide the following:

1. _____
2. _____
3. _____
4. _____

Of these, I will need help with the following from other sources (see Resource Directory for support agencies):

Source: _____

Source: _____

Source: _____

Source: _____

If and as I assume more responsibility for caring for my parents, I'm going to do the following for myself to ensure that I can cope most effectively:

_____
_____
_____
_____
_____
_____
_____
_____
_____

Notes:

_____
_____
_____
_____
_____
_____
_____
_____
_____
_____
_____
_____
_____
_____
_____
_____
_____
_____
_____

A FINANCIAL PRIMER:

Managing Your Parents' Finances

If you're going to help your parents evaluate their financial situation, or if you have to make financial decisions for them, there are some key steps to take and considerations to bear in mind.

To accurately determine your parents' financial status, you should first create two statements: a Net Worth Statement and an Income and Expenses Statement. Your parents' accountant should be helpful in this exercise.

When completed, the Net Worth Statement will show the current value of your parents' estate. Assets such as homes, investments, Registered Retirement Savings Plans, and pensions should be listed in this section. This statement also should show current liabilities, such as any mortgages or loans. Assets minus liabilities results in net worth. Taxes may have to be taken into consideration in the event that investments are sold. At the end of the calculation, you should know your parents' net worth in case you need to liquidate some or all of their holdings in order to provide for their care.

The Income and Expenses Statement will show your parents' sources of income and current expenses. This may include government benefits, such as Canada Pension Plan/Quebec Pension Plan benefits, Old Age Security benefits, and other provincial or federal income that your parents may be qualified to receive. Employer pension plans, private annuities, and Registered Retirement Income Fund payments also should be included, as well as income from bonds, Guaranteed Investment Certificates (GICs), or other investments. Once again, bear in mind that the income may be reduced by taxes. You should always have a copy of your parents' income tax return from the previous year. It'll outline all of the sources of income.

It's also a good idea to have copies of statements of your parents' investments. These statements will show the name of the company, the contract number, the name of the contact person or representative, and a list of the investments. Having copies of these at hand will save you a lot of trouble. Just make sure they're updated annually.

Many elderly people are in a high marginal tax bracket. This is because they generally invest in passive investments such as GICs or bonds that attract high tax rates.

INVESTMENTS

If your parents are concerned that they're paying too much in taxes, and if they have funds invested in GICs, there may be other financial vehicles that are more tax efficient and will generate income for them on a guaranteed basis. Financial instruments such as prescribed annuities generate income that is tax favourable, continue for life, and are guaranteed. The tax efficient prescribed annuity can also reduce the amount of old age security clawback while increasing income.

Segregated funds may also be appropriate for older individuals who want their capital to be protected. The capital of these funds is protected under federal regulation. Investments are varied and can be volatile; however, the segregated funds have a guaranteed death benefit. In other words, if an individual dies while holding a segregated fund, his or her capital is protected.

In some cases, both parents and children are concerned with relinquishing control of the capital to a company that issues annuities. However, an arrangement can be structured where a parent receives income for life in a tax efficient manner and then the capital is returned tax-free to his or her estate upon death.

Many elderly individuals invest in mutual funds. It's important for your parents' financial advisor to accurately measure their risk tolerance and their understanding of the volatility of the market. Unfortunately, many a nest egg has been lost because of misunderstanding and misinformation. If your parents aren't investment savvy, you may want to take an interest in their portfolio and sit in on the meetings with their advisors.

Long-Term Care Insurance

Long-term care insurance has recently been introduced in Canada. This form of insurance will become increasingly popular as the population ages. It's generally available to people until the age of eighty. A pre-existing health condition doesn't automatically exclude an individual from qualifying for this kind of insurance.

The long-term care insurance plan provides for either a daily or a monthly benefit to be used to supplement care needed at home or in a long-term care facility. In order to qualify for long-term care insurance, an individual must be able to perform at lease two out of the six daily living activities or be cognitively impaired.

This type of insurance plan can be designed to fit a person's ability to pay the premium. Benefits may be received for a designated number of years or for a lifetime, and the level of the monthly benefit can vary to suit an individual's needs and cash flow.

Today, many parents and their children are jointly subscribing for long-term care plans. By having a long-term care insurance plan in place, parents are ensured that they'll receive the necessary funding to live out their lives in comfort and dignity. As important, their children won't have to feel guilty if they can't financially provide for their parents in their time of need.

REVERSE MORTGAGE

A reverse mortgage is a financial tool through which individuals can free up equity in their home in order to generate an income, without selling the property. The older the individual and the higher the value of the property, the more can be borrowed. At death, or when the home is sold, the loan and the interest are repaid.

Psychologically, many people might have problems with assuming a mortgage in their later years. Also, it's possible with a reverse mortgage that when the house is sold, 100 percent of the proceeds will be needed to pay off the loan. This may marginalize or even wipe out any inheritance for heirs.

LIFE INSURANCE

Many older people never had, or have cancelled, their life insurance contract. This is unfortunate but it's not surprising. Years ago, the main purpose of life insurance was to protect the family if the wage earner died prematurely. It was also used in the event of death to pay off a mortgage. However, as children grew, many people no longer saw the need for their life insurance plan. Even if a parent can't afford the premiums on an existing life insurance policy, the child should consider paying the premium on behalf of the parent, because many of these policies accumulate cash value that can be used as collateral for a loan or to help generate income. As well, many older policies have tax efficient advantages, and the cash in the policies continues to grow in a tax-sheltered environment.

If, as a child, you need to provide financial support to your parents, a life insurance policy could be used to replace some of the money spent for care.

Even if your parents don't want to designate a child or their estate as beneficiary of the insurance policies, those policies still can be used in a tax efficient way by designating a charity as beneficiary. On death, the charity receives the cash benefit, and the estate receives a tax credit that can be used in the year of death or in the previous year to offset other taxes.

CRITICAL ILLNESS INSURANCE

Critical Illness Insurance is a relatively new insurance product. The plan insures an individual for a predetermined amount up to $2 million. If the person contracts one of the listed critical illnesses (there are about twenty-two illness covered in most contracts) and survives thirty days, the lump sum is paid to the survivor.

In most plans, if the insured dies without collecting a claim, all the premiums paid into the plan are refunded. The funds received from a critical illness insurance plan may be used to seek medical care, renovate a home, or take a vacation. How the money is used is not restricted in any way.

The cost of critical illness plans varies based on age of the client, amount of coverage, and the plan design.

EMPLOYER BENEFITS AND RETIREMENT INCOME

Most employer health plans don't provide retirement benefits. However, some do on a limited basis, while others might be more extensive. If your parents worked for a large company or for a government agency, they may have retirement benefits, including chronic care benefits. If they do, they're among the lucky few. Ask your parents if they have a copy of the Employee Health Benefit Booklet. If they don't have a copy, contact their past employers and check with the plan administrator.

Most pension plans pay out their employees in the form of a life or joint life annuity. This means a payment will continue for as long as either the employee and/or the spouse lives. There may be a guarantee period, defining the number of years that the payments are received. If the annuity is a joint life annuity, it'll continue for as long as either of your parents is alive. It's important that you know where the documents are located.

There are other forms of income that your parents may be receiving aside from annuities. Some are more flexible, in that the owner can determine the amount received and the nature of the investment. The cash flow may be increased in some cases (such as in a critical or palliative care situation) or decreased to preserve the capital and lower income tax. It's important that the family has a clear understanding of these contracts and their flexibility.

Travel Insurance

It's critical for the elderly to have travel insurance, especially if they plan to travel outside of their jurisdiction. The cost of medical care in the event of an emergency out of province can be astronomical. Before your parents travel outside of their province, you should be sure that they have appropriate protection in case of a health emergency. And remind them to carry their travel insurance certificate with them whenever outside of the province, while also leaving a copy with you or in a place to which you have easy access.

Pick the Right Financial Planner and Be Prepared

First and foremost, don't wait until it's too late. The sooner a family meets and plans together with their aging parents, the better. It's not easy, but if you think the time has come to become involved in your parents' financial planning, it probably has. Meet with them and find out if they've worked with a qualified financial planner. If they haven't, seek out a planner who has a proven understanding of — and experience in — the senior market. Ask around. A chartered financial consultant, a chartered life underwriter, a specialist in eldercare planning, or a chartered accountant who is part of Prime Plus will be able to help you and your parents.

If and when you meet a qualified financial planner, come prepared. Bring your parents' last will and testament, the power of attorney, a list of bank accounts, a list of investments, last year's income tax return, their accountant's and lawyer's names, addresses, and phone numbers, and the names of any other advisors.

Ask the planner to project the amount of income your parents would receive if they turn all their assets into income-generating investments. Discuss their investment risk tolerance. Review their health plan. Ask about tax efficient plans specifically designed for the elderly. Find out what is available from the government. Discuss long-term care plans.

Be prepared, be informed, and plan not for what might happen, but for what's likely to happen.

Resource Directory

One of the most difficult and time-consuming tasks you'll face when dealing with aging parents is identifying and finding the right resources that offer the information, help, and support your parents need — and that *you'll* need in order to help them. The hard part is knowing how to locate those resources and figuring out which ones offer what services or support mechanisms.

This updated resource directory is your guide to national and provincial/territorial contacts for advice and help. There are an amazing number of resources across Canada — many more, in fact, than just two years ago when we originally compiled the directory. There also are many different kinds of medical specialties available to help, and they are defined in this resource directory to help demystify them.

While the resource directory is comprehensive, it doesn't attempt to be definitive, and we've refrained from trying to identify the many local support groups that exist. For those, it's best to consult your regional health authority or local hospital, or even to speak with your parents' physician or your own. However, based on our research over the past number of months, we believe that this resource directory is one of the — if not the — most thorough compilations of its kind in Canada at this moment.

We've done the best we could to ensure the contact names, telephone numbers, and websites are current and accurate as of late 2004.

But as we discovered, phone numbers and websites are always being changed, so we're sorry for any inconvenience should you find an error.

As the challenge of caring for elderly parents continues to mushroom, there also are a growing number of local qualified individuals who — and smaller organizations that — can provide counsel and support.

These are often former social workers, nurses, and others who specialize in various aspects of eldercare support. Frankly, asking around is just about the best way to find them.

And finally, because so many of us are comfortable searching the Web for information and resources, a word of caution: beware of all those sites that freely offer advice and guidance; ensure that those sites are not only current but also qualified. That, of course, takes some time and assessment on your part: demanding, yes, yet also critical to ensure that what you embrace is correct and helpful to you and your parents.

FINDING THE INFORMATION YOU NEED

This guide contains contact information for many organizations and services, listed both by *geographical location* and by *category* or *type of service*. Many websites listed here will lead you to other interesting and useful organizations. If you're unable to find a particular listing for your province or territory, try referring to the same category in the Canada-wide listings. National associations or organizations will be able to direct you to their closest location.

TABLE OF CONTENTS

Your Guide to Health Professionals   286

Canada-wide   289

Alberta   303

British Columbia   313

Manitoba   321

New Brunswick   329

Newfoundland and Labrador   337

Northwest Territories   343

Nova Scotia   347

Nunavut   355

Ontario   359

Prince Edward Island   369

Quebec   375

Saskatchewan   381

Yukon   387

CATEGORIES

PROFESSIONAL SERVICES
Professional colleges and associations that refer caregivers to health care professionals in their area.

FEDERAL/PROVINCIAL/TERRITORIAL GOVERNMENT
Government agencies that help caregivers access relevant health care services.

LONG-TERM CARE FACILITIES
Facilities (public and private) that provide medical care to those who need it.

GENERAL RESOURCES
A collection of helpful services and associations to help you provide better care.

NURSING AND HOMEMAKING AGENCIES
Visiting nurses and homemakers that provide in-home assistance.

HOME HEALTH CARE RETAILERS, HOME SAFETY, AND ENVIRONMENT
Services and retailers that provide adaptive home equipment, alarms, renovations, and more.

FINANCIAL PLANNING/LEGAL
Organizations that will help with financial and legal matters.

DRIVING CAPABILITY ASSESSMENT
Provincial/territorial ministries and driving assessment programs.

SPECIAL NEEDS
Organizations that provide services for other medical conditions (e. g., the blind or deaf population).

CARING FOR YOURSELF
Counselling and support services for the caregiver.

Your Guide to Health Professionals

When it comes to caring for your parents, you're not alone. There are many qualified health care professionals ready to help, each with his or her own special expertise. Here's a quick introduction to the health professionals you may encounter in your caregiving journey.

OCCUPATIONAL THERAPIST

Occupational therapists focus on helping people be as engaged as possible in activities and occupations that are meaningful to them, based on the individual's abilities, needs, and interests. As a person becomes more dependent, the occupational therapist will continue to work collaboratively with you and other caregivers. They'll help to develop a safe and supportive environment that encourages your parents to participate in their lives as much as they are able by identifying and recommending customized solutions that could include modifying tasks and/or environments and using assistive devices such as wheelchairs and bathroom equipment. The therapist may help you to identify strategies to make sure that you are looking after your needs as well, in your role as the caregiver.

For more information, contact the Canadian Association of Occupational Therapists, 1-800-434-2268, http://www.caot.ca.

PHYSICIANS

Family Physician

Family physicians provide continuing and comprehensive general medical care, health maintenance and preventive services to individuals. They are involved in coordinating medical care.

The family physician will know your parents' medical condition. Because of the their familiarity with their patients, family physicians are best qualified to serve as an advocate in all health-related matters, including the appropriate use of consultants, health services, and community resources.

For more information, contact The College of Family Physicians of Canada, 1-800-387-6197, http://www.cfpc.ca.

Geriatrician

A geriatrician is a physician specially trained in the health needs and problems of the elderly. Most geriatricians are internists or family physicians certified in geriatric medicine. Family physicians and local hospitals are your best sources for finding the kind of geriatricians you may need.

Neurologist

A neurologist is a physician with specialized training in diagnosing, treating, and managing disorders of the brain and nervous system, including Alzheimer's disease. A neurologist will diagnose the condition, determine the proper treatment, and work with the family physician and others in managing a patient's overall health.

Psychiatrist/Geriatric Psychiatrist

A psychiatrist is able to diagnose and treat behavioural and emotional challenges that result from any form of dementia that may be emerging or that may have been present for some time. Psychiatrists are medical doctors with extra training in psychiatry and are thus able to prescribe medication for treatment.

Physiotherapist

Physiotherapists, also known as physical therapists, are health care professionals trained in the study of rehabilitation who evaluate, restore, and maintain physical function. They have a detailed understanding of how the body works and are trained to assess and improve movement and function and to relieve associated pain.

For more information, contact the Canadian Physiotherapy Association, 1-800-387-8679, http://www.physiotherapy.ca.

Psychologist

Psychologists specialize in treating behavioural, emotional, and motivational problems. They can assess cognitive dysfunctions and recommend non-drug treatments and intervention programs.

Psychologists who work with clients are sometimes called clinical psychologists. Neuropsychologists specialize in the diagnosis of brain disorders.

For more information, contact the Canadian Psychological Association, 1-613-237-2144, http://www.cpa.ca.

REGISTERED NURSES/REGISTERED PRACTICAL NURSES

Registered nurses and registered practical nurses are often involved in the care and treatment of persons with any health-related need. From providing direct clinical care in the home or hospital to providing information and counselling and helping to assess overall health needs, nursing professionals can help you to develop a comprehensive plan for care.

Nurses can help with medical and medication issues and can help you arrange for support services, such as home support, respite care, and day programs. Nurses work closely with physicians and are key members of the team. A registered nursing assistant or a home health aide may also provide in-home care under the direction of a registered nurse.

For more information, contact the Canadian Nursing Association, 1-800-361-8404, http://www.cna-nurses.ca.

SOCIAL WORKERS

Social workers help individuals, families, groups, and communities to resolve problems that affect their well-being on an individual or collective basis. They focus on the relationships between people and their environments, helping to enhance problem-solving and coping capacities.

For individuals and families coping with the challenge of aging parents, social workers offer counselling for crisis intervention when health and safety are at risk and for loss and grief. As well, they are able to help caregivers to access support services.

For more information, contact the Canadian Association of Social Workers, 1-613-729-6668, http://www.casw-acts.ca.

SPEECH-LANGUAGE PATHOLOGISTS/ AUDIOLOGISTS

These professionals specialize in speech, language, and hearing disorders. Speech-language pathologists help individuals overcome and prevent communication problems in language, speech, voice, and fluency. Audiologists assess the extent of any hearing loss, balance and related disorders, and recommend appropriate treatment.

For more information, contact the Canadian Association of Speech Language Pathologists and Audiologists, 1-800-259-8519, http://www.caslpa.ca.

CANADA-WIDE

FEDERAL GOVERNMENT

Reference Canada

Telephone: 1-800-622-6232; (TTY/TDD) 1-800-465-7735
Website: www.canada.gc.ca

A central source of information for all federal government programs and services. Telephone lines are staffed by information officers who will direct you to federal programs, information sources, and services.

Services for Seniors Guide

The federal government has issued a national guide, *Services for Seniors*, that covers everything from health, pensions, and taxes to recreation, volunteering, and the Internet. Copies are available in large print, audiotape, and Braille. To order, call 1-800-622-6232 or (TTY) 1-800-465-7735.

Health Canada, Division of Aging and Seniors

Telephone: 613-946-8043
Website: www.hc-sc.gc.ca/english/for_you/seniors.html

Provides information on a broad range of health-related issues. To receive publications, visit the website, call 613-952-7606, or send an email to seniors@hc-sc.gc.ca.

Human Resources and Skills Development Canada

Telephone: (English) 1-800-277-9914; (French) 1-800-277-9915;
(TTY) 1-800-255-4786
Website: www.hrsdc.gc.ca/en

HRSDC administers two income assistance programs for seniors (Canada Pension Plan and Old Age Security) through its Income Security Programs. For information, call the appropriate 1-800 number above or visit the website.

Canadian Seniors Policies and Programs Database

Website: www.sppd.gc.ca; Email: sppd-bdppa@hc-sc.gc.ca

The SPPD is a very helpful Internet-based database of government policies and programs for which seniors are the primary beneficiaries. It was developed and is maintained by federal, provincial, and territorial governments. Select your province or territory from the menu.

Seniors Canada On-line

Website: www.seniors.gc.ca

Seniors Canada On-line provides single-window access to Web-based information and services that are relevant to seniors 55+, their families, caregivers, and supporting service organizations. This is an exceptionally helpful website. Links are provided to information on a wide range of subjects such as safe driving courses, home care, health, housing, calculating Old Age Security payments, food and nutrition, and sexuality, as well as to the weather, Canada 411, and Canada Post's postal code lookup. Start your search for Web-based seniors' information here.

Veterans Affairs Canada

Telephone: (English) 1-866-522-2122; (French) 1-866-522-2022
Website: www.vac-acc.gc.ca; Email: information@vac-acc.gc.ca

The Veterans Independence Program provides special home care services to Canadian veterans. Services range from transportation, home adaptations, counselling, and health care to house cleaning and maintenance. There are income qualifications for specific services. Call the number above to find the regional office nearest you.

GENERAL RESOURCES

Alzheimer Society of Canada

Telephone: 1-800-616-8816
Website: www.alzheimer.ca; Email: info@alzheimer.ca

The Alzheimer Society provides a nationwide network of support and helps people find programs and services (day and respite programs, home support, and help with the difficult transition to long-term care), administers a nationwide Alzheimer Wandering Registry, and offers many educational tools and resources for caregivers.

Arthritis Society

Telephone: 1-800-321-1433
Website: www.arthritis.ca

A non-profit organization devoted to funding and promoting arthritis research, patient care, and public education. There are divisions in each province; see the provincial listings for details.

Canadian Cancer Society

Cancer Information Service: 1-888-939-3333
Website: www.cancer.ca; Email: ccs@cancer.ca
For information about cancer: info@cis.cancer.ca

The toll-free line is a good entry point for those with questions and to learn the telephone number of your local divisional office. Each office provides various kinds of support and services. The website has a number of informative articles that you can download, as well as access to *The Canadian Cancer Encyclopedia*, a comprehensive, searchable database of cancer information. Another useful feature is found by clicking on "Cancer Information" at the top of the page to read short definitions of many types of cancer.

Canadian Council of the Blind

Telephone: 613-567-0311 or 1-877-304-0968
Website: www.ccbnational.net; Email: ccb@national.net

A national self-help consumer organization of people who are blind and deaf-blind. Contact the national office for services in your area.

Canadian Deafblind & Rubella Association

Telephone: 519-754-0729
Website: www.cdbra.ca; Email: cdbra.nat@sympatico.ca

Provides intervention services to deaf-blind and rubella handicapped people across Canada. To locate the provincial chapters, call the number above or visit the website.

Canadian Diabetes Association

Telephone: 416-363-0177 or 1-800-BANTING (226-8464)
Website: www.diabetes.ca; Email: info@diabetes.ca

With more than 150 branches across Canada, the Canadian Diabetes Association supports research, education, and advocacy for and on behalf of those with various levels of diabetes. The helpful website provides information to patients and professionals; patient information is available in English and Chinese.

Canadian Health Network

Website: www.canadian-health-network.ca

CHN is a national Internet-based health information service with links to some 10,000 health-related resources. On the home page of the website, under the heading "Groups," click on "Seniors" for the section dedicated to the health information needs of Canadians 65 years and older.

Canadian Hearing Society

Telephone: 416-928-2500 or 1-877-347-3427;
(TTY) 416-964-0023 or 1-877-347-3429
Website: www.chs.ca; Email: info@chs.ca

The Canadian Hearing Society provides services and programs that encourage prevention of hearing loss and enhance the independence of deaf, deafened, and hard of hearing people. Several programs are provided, including a hearing aid program to dispense and fit hearing aids and a hearing care counselling program for those 55 years and older. There is a comprehensive cross-Canada directory of resources on the website at www.chs.ca/pdf/Contacts%20in%20Canada.pdf. Call one of the numbers above or send an email to be referred to the office nearest you.

Canadian Home Care Association

Telephone: 613-569-1585
Website: www.cdnhomecare.ca

The CHCA focuses on the advancement of quality home and community care nationally through information and knowledge sharing in order to facilitate best practices at all levels. On the website, the "Related Sites" tab has helpful links to several Canadian caregiver and health information websites.

Canadian Mental Health Association

Telephone: 416-484-7750
Website: www.cmha.ca; Email: info@cmha.ca

The CMHA focuses on combatting mental health problems and emotional disorders through more than 10,000 volunteers and staff in 135 branches across Canada.

Canadian National Institute for the Blind

Telephone: 416-486-2500
Website: www.cnib.ca

The CNIB is a national volunteer agency that provides a range of services to those suffering from varying degrees of loss of vision, with offices across Canada. It offers numerous resources, including counselling and referral, orientation and mobility training, sight enhancement, and technical aids.

Canadian Red Cross Society

Telephone: (National office) 613-740-1900; (Atlantic region) 506-674-6200; (Ontario region) 905-890-1000; (Quebec region) 514-362-2930; (Western region) 403-205-3448
Website: www.redcross.ca

The Canadian Red Cross provides a number of home care services and equipment loans for eligible persons. One example is the Home Support Service: a complete program of in-home care services. Services vary by region; call your regional office to find specific services offered in your area.

The Complete Aging and Caregiving Resource Guide

Website: www.caregiver.on.ca/resource.pdf

Developed from the television program *Caregiving with June Callwood*, this is a very thorough listing of federal and provincial resources and services available to those who are providing care for a parent, spouse, or themselves. You will need Adobe Acrobat to view this document. You can download a free copy at www.adobe.com/products/acrobat/readstep2.html.

Heart and Stroke Foundation of Canada

Telephone: 613-569-4361
Website: www.heartandstroke.ca

This organization has more than 250,000 volunteers dedicated to improving health by preventing and reducing disability and death from heart disease. You can access provincial websites by selecting a province from the drop-down menu on the left side of the home page.

Meals on Wheels

This program provides hot meals delivered to seniors in their homes. There are hundreds of Meals on Wheels programs across Canada. To find the program nearest you, please check your local phone directory or ask your care coordinator or family physician.

Medbroadcast Corporation

Website: www.medbroadcast.com

This Vancouver-based company specializes in providing online consumer health and wellness information and services. Click on "Senior's health" on the left side of the page. The website also contains very useful information on Canadian prescription drugs. Click on the "Drugs" tab at the top of the page.

Internet Mental Health

Website: www.mentalhealth.com

Internet Mental Health is a free encyclopedia of mental health information created by Canadian psychiatrist Dr. Phillip Long.

Salvation Army

Telephone: 416-425-2111
Website: www.salvationarmy.ca

The Salvation Army provides pastoral care visits upon request. It also operates some long-term care facilities, respite care programs, and day-away programs in co-operation with local health care authorities. Services vary from region to region.

SeniorsCan

Website: www.crm.mb.ca

The SeniorsCan Internet Program is a highly acclaimed guide for retirees and older adults to Canadian and global information and services. There is a very useful listing of services and contacts for each province. On the home page, click on "Canada by Province," then click on the flag for your province.

NURSING AND HOMEMAKING AGENCIES

Both non-profit and private nursing agencies provide nursing and support personnel to clients in their homes. A case manager/care coordinator from your regional health authority, local Community Care Access Centre, or Centres Locaux de Service Communitaires will provide a needs assessment to determine if funding is available.

A variety of funded services are available, including nursing, homemaking, respite, and personal care. For example, personal support workers are often provided for people with physical disabilities, advancing dementia, or Alzheimer's to help with household chores and/or personal care.

You can also purchase extra help by contacting a local nursing or homemaking agency directly and arranging to pay for the services you need to supplement those paid for by the government. Ask your health professional for names of local agencies to contact.

Bayshore Health Care
Telephone: 1-800-461-5586
Website: www.bayshore.ca; Email: info@bayshore.ca
A private nursing agency with a full range of nursing and homemaking services.

Caregivers.ca
Telephone: 416-788-CARE (2273)
Website: www.caregivers.ca; Email: home@caregivers.ca
This private firm helps families find caregivers from dozens of countries and arranges all related immigration matters.

Comcare Health Services
Telephone: 1-800-663-5775
Website: www.comcarehealth.ca
A private nursing agency with a full range of nursing and homemaking services. Call the number above or visit the website to find the office nearest you.

ParaMed Home Health Care
Telephone: 1-800-465-5054
Website: www.extendicare.com
A private nursing agency with a full range of home healthcare services. Call the number above or visit the website and click on "Services & Locations" for details.

Extendicare (Canada) Inc.
Telephone: 905-470-4000
Website: www.extendicare.com

One of North America's largest operators of long-term care facilities, Extendicare has facilities across most of Canada.

Victorian Order of Nurses (VON)

Telephone: 613-233-5694

Website: www.von.ca; Email: national@von.ca

A non-profit agency. In addition to traditional nursing services, most provincial branches of the VON provide day-away programs for persons with dementia. These programs give caregivers a break while providing their clients with an opportunity to socialize and maintain their independence. Call the number above or visit the website to find the office nearest you.

We Care Home Health Care Services

Telephone: 416-922-7601 or 1-888-429-3227

Website: www.wecare.ca

A private agency offering franchised nursing and homemaking services across Canada. Call the number above or visit the website to find the office nearest you.

HOME HEALTH CARE RETAILERS, HOME SAFETY AND ENVIRONMENT

A variety of home health care products and services are available from national retailers and also from your local pharmacy. Depending on your location, many stores offer in-home assessments, equipment trials, and rental programs for short-term needs.

Your health professional should be able to refer you to local stores, or you can call and ask one of the following national retailers for the location closest to your home.

As well, there are government support programs and a Canada Post alert program that are worth exploring as the need arises.

Canada Mortgage and Housing Corporation (CMHC)

Telephone: 1-800-668-2642

Website: www.cmhc.ca; Email: chic@cmhc-schl.gc.ca

CMHC's Home Adaptations for Seniors' Independence (HASI) program is designed to provide information about and fund home adaptations related to accessibility for seniors 65 and over. A forgiveable loan of up to $3,500 is provided to qualified applicants (based on gross household income) for fixed items such as ramps, stair glides, and grab bars. Its Residential Rehabilitation Assistance Program (RRAP) offers differing levels of financial assistance for homeowners and landlords who are modifying dwellings for occupancy by low-income persons with disabilities.

The programs are administered on a provincial or municipal level depending on the region. In some areas, there is supplemental funding available from the province as well.

Canada Post's Letter Carriers Alert Program

Telephone: 1-800-267-1177
Website: www.canadapost.ca

Canada Post's letter carriers keep an eye on customers and report if they detect an unusual build-up of mail or newspapers at the customers' residences. This service is free in participating communities. Contact your local postmaster or call the toll-free number and ask a customer service representative if there is a program in your area.

Canadian MedicAlert Foundation

Telephone: (English) 1-800-668-1507; (French) 1-800-668-6381
Website: www.medicalert.ca; Email: medinfo@medicalert.ca

The Canadian MedicAlert Foundation provides service and protection to Canadians with medical information and personal requests that should be known in the event of a medical emergency, including medical conditions, drug and food allergies, special needs, and medications.

Lifecall of Canada

Telephone: 1-800-661-5433
Website: www.lifecall.ca; Email: customer.support@voxcom.com

Lifecall is an emergency response service that provides immediate attention to seniors in need. It can offer peace of mind for caregivers and family members; however, seniors must remember to use the service. There is a fee.

Lifeline Systems Canada Inc.

Telephone: 1-800-543-3546
Website: www.lifeline.ca

Personal response service for people living alone or at risk. A portable alarm button is linked by telephone line to a central call centre. A fee is charged.

MEDIchair

Telephone: 1-800-667-0087
Website: www.medichair.com; Email: medichair@medichair.com

There are MEDIchair locations from coast to coast providing a full range of medical equipment for assisted daily living.

Motion Group

Telephone: 1-800-267-2920
Website: www.themotiongroup.com; Email: msinfo@themotiongroup.com

More than 30 specialized providers of seating, patient room equipment, mobility products, and assistive devices for persons with disabilities.

Shoppers HomeHealthCare

Telephone: 1-800-746-7737
Website: www.shoppersdrugmart.ca;
Email: customerservice@shoppersdrugmart.ca

A network of specialized stores that offer a wide variety of home health care and wellness products for safety, comfort, and independence. Professionally trained staff work with you to assess your needs. Home visits are available without charge.

FINANCIAL PLANNING/LEGAL

The following organizations will refer you to trained professionals in your region who will assist you with general information you may need and on various aspects of estate and financial planning as well as protecting your rights.

Canada Revenue Agency

Telephone: 1-800-959-8281
Website: www.ccra-adrc.gc.ca

This is the government agency responsible for all tax matters within Canada. It maintains taxation records as well as information on the Canada Pension Plan.

Canadian Institute of Chartered Accountants

Telephone: 416-977-8585 or 1-800-268-3793
Website: www.cica.ca

The Institute will provide a listing of accounting firms by geographical information and has a subsection called "Prime Plus" that designates firms that, and accountants who, specialize in meeting the financial planning needs of the elderly.

Certified General Accountants Association of Canada

Telephone: 1-800-663-1529

Website: www.cga-canada.org; Email: public@cga-canada.org

This group will refer you to your provincial association, which will, in turn, provide a list of accountants within a local area. Call the above number, send an email, or go to the website and click on "CGA Affiliates."

Financial Advisors Association of Canada — Advocis

Telephone: 1-800-563-5822

Website: www.advocis.ca; Email: info@advocis.ca

This organization represents professionals who can provide assistance with overall financial planning. Look on the website to find a financial planner; click on "Find an advisor" at the top of the page.

Operation Phone Busters

Telephone: 1-888-495-8501

Website: www.phonebusters.com; Email: info@phonebusters.com

A free national telephone service that helps fight telemarketing fraud. Offers free video information tapes and pamphlets.

SPECIAL NEEDS

The associations and foundations below offer a wealth of information and contacts on specific conditions other than dementia.

Aphasia Institute

Telephone: 416-226-3636

Website: www.aphasia.ca; Email: aphasia@aphasia.ca

The Aphasia Institute helps those with a language disorder resulting from an injury to the brain — most often a stroke. Offers direct services in the Greater Toronto Area but can help with training and communications resources across Canada.

Canadian Association of the Deaf

Telephone: 613-565-2882; (TTY) 613-565-8882
Website: www.cad.ca; Email: cad@cad.ca

A national consumer group that provides a research and information centre, a self-help society, and a community action organization.

Canadian Continence Foundation

Telephone: 1-800-265-9575
Website: www.continence-fdn.ca; Email: help@continence-fdn.ca

The Canadian Continence Foundation offers a wealth of information on incontinence management and treatment, including books, videos, audiotapes, and newsletters. The Foundation also will put you in touch with health care professionals who have expertise with urinary incontinence.

Canadian Hard of Hearing Association

Telephone: 1-800-263-8068
Website: www.chha.ca

The CHHA provides information and brochures on improving communication skills and helping people deal with hearing loss. There is a seniors' manual with helpful advice available for $4.00 per copy.

Canadian National Society of the Deaf-Blind

Telephone: n/a; Fax: 416-223-0182
Website: www.cnsdb.ca; Email: cnsdb@canada.com

The Society distributes information to help the deaf-blind and those who are caring for them.

Canadian Hospice Palliative Care Association

Telephone: 1-800-668-2785;
(Hospice Palliative Care Info Line) 1-877-203-4636
Website: www.chpca.net; Email: info@chpca.net

The Association provides leadership in hospice palliative care, which is aimed at relief of suffering, loneliness, and grief for those who are approaching death.

Dietitians of Canada

Telephone: 416-596-0857
Website: www.dietitians.ca

Dietitians provide tips on nutrition and eating management. The organization doesn't provide names over the phone; however, you can visit the website and search for a local dietitian in your area.

Dying with Dignity

Telephone: 1-800-495-6156
Website: www.dyingwithdignity.ca; Email: info@dyingwithdignity.ca

This organization educates caregivers on the rights of their loved ones as they near the end of life. They also provide counselling and information on living wills, advance health care directives, and power of attorney. They can refer caregivers to a local health care professional with specialized training in end-of-life care.

Osteoporosis Society of Canada

Telephone: (English) 1-800-463-6842; (French) 1-800-977-1778
Website: www.osteoporosis.ca; Email: osc@osteoporosis.ca

The Society assists people who have osteoporosis and those who are at risk. Services include free publications, a bilingual toll-free information line, educational programs, and referrals to self-help groups and community resources. Visit the website or call the number above to find the chapter nearest you.

Tetra Society of North America

Telephone: 604-688-6464 or 1-877-688-8762
Website: www.tetrasociety.org; Email: info@tetrasociety.org

The Tetra Society matches community volunteers with people with special needs. These volunteers then create custom-designed assistive devices to help improve the individual's daily life. Visit the website or call the number above to find the chapter nearest you.

CARING FOR YOURSELF

Canada's Association for the Fifty-Plus

Telephone: 416-363-8748 or 1-800-363-9736
Website: www.50plus.com; Email: carp@50plus.com

A national association for those 50 and older that provides a range of services, including advice on health, travel, and finances. Links on the website take you to useful sites such as the Canada Pension Plan, Old Age Security, and the Passport Office. Free electronic newsletters are available on a variety of topics. Group savings are available on a range of benefits, including insurance, travel, and car rental. Membership is free.

The Canadian Caregiver Coalition

Telephone: 1-888-866-2273
Website: www.ccc-ccan.ca; Email: ccc_ccan@von.ca

This is an alliance of individuals, groups, and organizations that promotes awareness and action to influence policy and address the needs of caregivers of all ages across Canada.

Caregiver Network Inc. (CNI)

Telephone: 416-323-1090
Website: www.caregiver.on.ca; Email: karenh@caregiver.on.ca

Although it is based in Toronto, the goal of CNI is to be a national single information source to make your life as a caregiver easier. The website has very helpful information on many topics of interest to caregivers, such as nutrition, support groups, driving, long-distance caregiving, and home care. There are also several useful links, for example, to the Alzheimer Society and the Canadian MedicAlert Foundation and sites that will help you locate home care services and housing.

Family Caregiver Alliance

Telephone: 415-434-3388
Website: www.caregiver.org; Email: info@caregiver.org

An American website with interesting information for family caregivers.

Solutions — Eldercare and Family Caregiving

Telephone: 1-866-290-2909
Website: www.solutions-online.ca

This magazine is published six times a year and positions itself as Canada's family guide to home health care and wellness. It provides readers with a host of tips and tactics on the challenges of caring for aging parents, as well as product and literature reviews.

ALBERTA

GOVERNMENT

For a full list of programs and services offered by the federal government, please refer to FEDERAL GOVERNMENT in the Canada-wide listings.

Toll-Free Access to All Provincial Government Programs

You can contact any provincial government program toll-free from anywhere in the province by calling Alberta's RITE line telephone service. Simply dial 310-0000 and then enter the telephone number you need or press zero for RITE assistance. If you do not have a touch-tone telephone, stay on the line and an operator will help you place your call.

Alberta Seniors Information Line and Seniors Service Centres

Telephone: 1-800-642-3853; (Edmonton) 780-427-7876; (TDD/TTY toll-free) 1-800-232-7215; (TDD/TTY in Edmonton) 780-427-9999
Website: www.seniors.gov.ab.ca

The toll-free Alberta Seniors Information Line and Seniors Service Centres offer comprehensive information on programs and services for seniors in Alberta. Additional information is listed in the Seniors Programs and Services Information Guide. Go to www.seniors.gov.ab.ca/publications and click on the title. You need Adobe Acrobat to read this document; there is a link to a free copy of Acrobat on the website. You can also get a copy by contacting the Alberta Seniors Information Line at the numbers above.

Regional Health Authorities

Telephone: for toll-free, dial 310-0000, then 780-427-1432
Website: www.health.gov.ab.ca/regions

In Alberta, any one of the nine regional health authorities is a good point of entry to the health care system. Your local health authority will conduct an assessment and direct you to the resources you need. In addition, there are a number of independent associations and organizations (such as nursing agencies) that contract work through the health authority. You may be able to access these private services directly and pay for any additional care you require.

Alberta Health and Wellness

Telephone: for toll-free, dial 310-0000, then 780-427-1432
Website: www.health.gov.ab.ca; Email: health.ahinform@gov.ab.ca.

This department provides information on provincial health services and departments related to home care and caring for people's special needs.

Alberta Seniors Housing Services Division

Telephone: for toll-free, dial 310-0000, then 780-422-0122 (Edmonton)
or 403-297-7453 (Calgary)
Website: www.seniors.gov.ab.ca/housing; Email: housing@gov.ab.ca

Facilitates the provision of adequate and affordable housing to seniors in need.

Home Support Alberta

Telephone: 403-423-2831

Twenty offices throughout the province provide a variety of home support services. Call for contact information for your local office.

LONG-TERM CARE FACILITIES

There are a number of facilities throughout the province that provide varying levels of care. Your local regional health authority has a complete list. Your care coordinator will be able to direct you to the proper facility based on the level of care your parents may need. You also can contact the Alberta Long Term Care Association, whose members represent the public, private, and voluntary sectors in the province; call 780-435-0699 in Edmonton, or 1-888-212-4581, or go to www.longtermcare.ab.ca. Email: info@longtermcare.ab.ca.

The Care Guide, Alberta Edition

Telephone: 1-800-311-2273
Website: www.thecareguide.com

Operated by CARE Planning Partners Inc., this site provides information on seniors' housing and care services. The site features provider search tools, community bulletin boards, and an online assessment tool. A print copy of its directory is available from the website or by calling the above number.

GENERAL RESOURCES

Alberta Council on Aging

Telephone: 780-423-9666 or 1-888-423-9666

Website: www.seniorfriendly.ca; Email: acaging@interbaun.com

A province-wide charitable organization concerned with the process of aging.

Alberta Association for Community Living

Telephone: 1-800-252-7556;

(Edmonton) 780-451-3055; (Calgary) 403-717-0361

Website: www.aacl.org

This organization helps aging individuals with developmental disabilities. Support services and counselling are based on need.

Alzheimer Society of Alberta and Northwest Territories

Telephone: 403-250-1303 or 1-888-233-0332

Website: www.alzheimer.ab.ca; Email: bshima@alzheimer.ab.ca

The Alzheimer Society provides educational and support programs to improve awareness and to assist families and individuals coping with the disease. The resource centre is open to the public. It can provide referrals to support groups in your local area and will mail information. Check the website or call the 1-888 number to find the chapter nearest you.

Arthritis Society, Alberta & Northwest Territories Division

Telephone: 403-228-2571 or 1-800-321-1433

Website: www.arthritis.ca; Email: info@ab.arthritis.ca

A non-profit organization devoted to funding and promoting arthritis research, patient care, and public education. Check the website or call the toll-free number to get the details on the offices and services nearest you.

Canadian Cancer Society, Alberta NWT Division

Telephone: 403-228-4487 or 1-888-661-2262
Cancer Information Services: 1-888-939-3333
Website: www.cancer.ab.ca; Email: info@cancer.ab.ca
For information about cancer: info@cis.cancer.ca

Each divisional office provides various kinds of support and advice; call to find out what is available.

Canadian Deafblind and Rubella Association (Alberta)

Telephone: 403-458-7790
Website: www.deafblindalberta.ca

Provides intervention services to deaf-blind and rubella handicapped people throughout Alberta.

Canadian Diabetes Association, Alberta & NWT Regions

Telephone: (Northern Alberta and NWT) 780-423-1232 or 1-800-563-0032;
(Southern Alberta) 403-266-0620
Website: www.diabetes.ca; Email: (Northern Alberta and NWT)
freda.badry@diabetes.ca or (Southern Alberta) karen.caughey@diabetes.ca

A national, independent, self-financing organization that works to improve the quality of life of Canadians affected by diabetes by being the leading force in research, service, advocacy, and education. A very helpful website provides information to patients and professionals; patient information is available in English and Chinese. Call the appropriate number above to find the office nearest you.

Canadian Hard of Hearing Association, Calgary Branch

Telephone: (Voice) 403-276-5080
Website: www.chha.ca; Email: ctudhope@telus.net

The association provides information and brochures on improving communication skills and helping people deal with hearing loss. Check the website or call the national office at 1-800-263-8068 or (TTY) 613-526-2692 for the branch nearest you.

Canadian Mental Health Association, Alberta Division

Telephone: 780-482-6576

Website: www.cmha.ab.ca; Email: division@cmha.ab.ca

The CMHA promotes the mental health of all people and serves mental health consumers, their families, and friends. See the website or call the number above to find the branch nearest you.

Canadian National Institute for the Blind, Alberta-NWT-Nunavut Division

Telephone: 403-488-4871

Website: www.cnib.ca/divisions/alberta; Email: alberta@cnib.ca

A charitable, non-profit agency that provides rehabilitation and support services to people who are blind or visually impaired. Call the number above or visit the website to find the office nearest you.

Canadian Red Cross Society

Telephone: (Southern Alberta) 403-541-6100;

(Northern Alberta) 780-423-2680

Website: www.redcross.ca

Offers a variety of services to seniors throughout the province, including homecare, meals on wheels, equipment loan programs, and a unique home partner program. Call for services in your area.

Heart and Stroke Foundation of Alberta, NWT and Nunavut

Telephone: 403-264-5549 or 1-888-473-4636

Website: www.heartandstroke.ca

Provides free literature on a wide range of topics such as controlling stress and cholesterol, managing high blood pressure, and smoking cessation. Call the 1-888 number above or visit the website to find the office nearest you.

Multiple Sclerosis Society of Canada, Alberta Division

Telephone: 780-463-1190 or 1-800-268-7582

Website: www.mssociety.ca/alberta; Email: info.alberta@mssociety.ca

Undertakes research into the cause and cure of multiple sclerosis and works to educate the public about the condition.

SeniorsCan Alberta Information

Website: www.crm.mb.ca/ab

The SeniorsCan Internet Program is a highly acclaimed guide for retirees and older adults to Canadian and global information and services. This is a very useful website for Alberta information.

NURSING AND HOMEMAKING AGENCIES

For nursing and homemaking agencies in your area, please refer to NURSING AND HOMEMAKING AGENCIES in the Canada-wide listings.

HOME HEALTH CARE RETAILERS, HOME SAFETY AND ENVIRONMENT

There are a number of home health care retailers located throughout the province that can help you find the right products for your specific needs. To find a store near you, please refer to HOME HEALTH CARE RETAILERS, HOME SAFETY, AND ENVIRONMENT in the Canada-wide listings.

Canada Mortgage and Housing Corporation, Prairie, Nunavut and Northwest Territories Division

Telephone: 403-515-3000; (TTY) 1-888-841-4975

Website: www.cmhc.ca

See the Canada-wide listing under HOME HEALTH CARE RETAILERS, HOME SAFETY, AND ENVIRONMENT for services offered. Visit the website or call the above number to find the office nearest you.

FINANCIAL PLANNING/LEGAL

ABCs of Fraud Program

Telephone: 604-437-1940 or 1-866-437-1940

Website: www.bcceas.ca/fraud2.shtml; Email: ceas@telus.net

This program provides group presentations in major centres across the country to educate seniors about fraud, distributes complimentary support materials, and provides referrals to additional resources. To book a presentation in Calgary, call the 1-866 number above.

Public Trustee of Alberta

Telephone: 780-427-2744 or 403-297-6541

Website: www.justice.gov.ab.ca/dependent_adults

This office is responsible for protecting the financial rights of cognitively challenged people. The staff help individuals make decisions on personal care and medical treatment. The office also advises family members on guardianship and on how to obtain the legal authority to make decisions on behalf of loved ones. The website is very useful for answering basic questions concerning trusteeship of dependent adults.

DRIVING CAPABILITY ASSESSMENT

In each province, the Ministry of Transportation makes the official decision on when a person must stop driving. The family physician is legally required to report any cases in which someone's driving ability may be impaired due to the progression of age or any resulting condition. The physician must file his or her report with a medical review board, which may, based on research and interviews with key health care professionals, request a driving assessment to determine driving skills. Based on test results, a decision will be made on whether the individual is allowed to drive.

If you are concerned about your parents' ability to drive, you can request an independent assessment. Such assessments, which are provided by private companies for a fee, will help you determine your parents' safety while on the road.

Alberta Transportation, Alberta Traffic Safety Initiative

Telephone: 780-422-8839 or for toll-free, dial 310-0000, then 422-8830

Website: www.saferoads.com/drivers/drivers/aging.html

This department provides driver assessments to determine driving competence. There is a very informative sheet entitled *Tips for Senior Drivers* at: www.saferoads.com/drivers/drivers/seniortips/seniortips.html.

DriveAble Testing

Telephone: 403-252-2243 or 1-877-433-1494

Website: www.driveable.com; Email: info@driveable.com

Driver assessment program for people with possible cognitive impairment. Fee for service. Call the 1-877 number above for the testing centre nearest you.

SPECIAL NEEDS

The Support Network: Edmonton's Crisis & Information Centre

Distress Line: (Edmonton and area) 780-482-HELP (4357); (Drayton Valley, High Prairie, and Westview and Aspen Health Authorities regions) 1-800-232-7288

A 24-hour, confidential, non-judgmental listening service that provides support and referrals for people experiencing difficulty in their lives. Help is also provided in suicide and violent situations.

Senior Abuse Help Line

Telephone: 780-454-8888

This is a 24-hour help line. Call for information about senior abuse or if you think a senior is being abused or taken advantage of.

CARING FOR YOURSELF

Calgary Health Region Family Caregiver Centre

Telephone: 403-303-6027

Website: www.familycaregivers.ab.ca;

Email: family.caregivers@calgaryhealthregion.ca

The centre refers unpaid caregivers to information and support services in the health system and the community. There are also a number of resources available such as books, videos, articles, educational workshops, and personalized resource kits to fit your situation.

The Family Centre of Northern Alberta

Telephone: 780-423-2831

A non-profit centre offering homemaking services for in-home care and appointments. Family counselling and development workshops/seminars and interpreting services are offered. Charges a sliding scale fee for services.

LOCAL INFORMATION CENTRES

In addition to Public Health Services and Family and Community Support Services offices, many communities have local information centres that provide information on the services available in your community. Larger centres are as follows:

Calgary: Kerby Centre

Telephone: 403-265-0661

Website: www.kerbycentre.com; Email: kerbycentre@kerbycentre.com

Calgary: Calgary Seniors Resource Society

Telephone: 403-266-6200

Edmonton: The Support Network Community Referral Line

Telephone: 780-482-4636

Website: www.thesupportnetwork.com; Email: csrl@thesupportnetwork.com

BRITISH COLUMBIA

GOVERNMENT

For a full list of programs and services offered by the federal government, please refer to FEDERAL GOVERNMENT in the Canada-wide listings.

There are a variety of non-profit and private organizations contracted through British Columbia's regional health authorities that can provide home support services. They range from minimal home care to homemaking and full-time, live-in care. They also offer supervision, respite, and personal support for persons with dementia.

The B.C. Ministry of Health Services can direct you to the regional health authority in your area; call the ministry's information line at 1-800-465-4911 or visit its website at www.healthservices.gov.bc.ca/socsec/contacts.html. For general information, call 250-952-1742 or visit www.healthservices.gov.bc.ca/bchealthcare.

Office for Seniors
Telephone: 250-952-1742 or 1-800-465-4911
Website: www.hlth.gov.bc.ca/seniors

Responsible for informing the public on government policies and programs for seniors. The *Information for Seniors* guide is available online on the home page by clicking on the title, or at www.hlth.gov.bc.ca/seniors/publications/infoforseniors.pdf. This is a comprehensive guide to programs and benefits in British Columbia.

LONG-TERM CARE FACILITIES

In British Columbia, long-term care is offered at extended care facilities throughout the province. Each facility has a specific number of multi-level care beds that offer varying levels of care. The first step is to call your local regional health authority and request an assessment. The assessment will help determine the level of care your parents require and any other needs. Admission to a facility is based on this assessment.

To locate your local regional health authority, call the B.C. Ministry of Health information line at 1-800-465-4911 or go to www.healthservices.gov.bc.ca/socsec/contacts.html.

The Care Guide, British Columbia Edition

Telephone: 1-800-311-2273

Website: www.thecareguide.com

Operated by CARE Planning Partners Inc., this site provides information on seniors' housing and care services. The site features provider search tools, community bulletin boards, and an online assessment tool. A print copy of its directory is available online or by calling the above number.

GENERAL RESOURCES/SPECIAL NEEDS

Alzheimer Society of British Columbia

Telephone: 604- 681-6530 or 1-800-667-3742

Website: www.alzheimerbc.org; Email: info@alzheimerbc.org

The Alzheimer Society provides educational and support programs to improve awareness and assist families and individuals coping with the disease. The society offers telephone support for families and caregivers throughout the province. Regional representatives, respite managers, and volunteers can be contacted by phone or by visiting a regional resource centre. An information package with more local material and a comprehensive facilities list can be requested at no charge.

The British Columbia Aphasia Centre

Telephone: 604-877-8066

Website: www.bcaphasia.org; Email: bcaphasia@telus.net

Supports those with speech and language difficulties usually associated with strokes.

Arthritis Society, BC & Yukon Division

Telephone: 604-714-5550 or 1-800-321-1433

Website: www.arthritis.ca/bc; Email: info@bc.arthritis.ca

A non-profit organization devoted to funding and promoting arthritis research, patient care, and public education. Check the website or call the toll-free number above to find the offices and services nearest you.

Canadian Cancer Society, BC & Yukon Division

Telephone: 604-872-4400 or 1-800-663-2524

Cancer Information Service: 1-888-939-3333

Website: www.bc.cancer.ca; General email: inquiries@bc.cancer.ca

For information about cancer: info@cis.cancer.ca

Each division office provides various kinds of support and advice; call to find out what is available.

Canadian Deafblind & Rubella Association, British Columbia Chapter

Telephone: 604-436-1882

Website: www.cdbra.ca; Email: wylie@telus.net

Provides intervention services to deaf-blind and rubella handicapped people throughout British Columbia.

Canadian Diabetes Association, BC and Yukon

Telephone: 604-732-1331 or 1-800-665-6526

Website: www.diabetes.ca; Email: infobc@diabetes.ca

A national, independent, self-financing organization that works to improve the quality of life of Canadians affected by diabetes by being the leading force in research, service, advocacy, and education. A very helpful website provides information to patients and professionals; patient information is available in English and Chinese. Call the number above for the local office nearest you.

Canadian Hard of Hearing Association, BC Chapter

Telephone: 1-866-888-2442

Website: www.chha-bc.org; Email chha_bc@yahoo.ca

Provides information and brochures on improving communication skills and helping people deal with hearing loss.

Canadian National Institute for the Blind, British Columbia-Yukon Division

Telephone: 604-431-2020

Website: www.cnib.ca/divisions/bc_yukon

A charitable, non-profit, voluntary agency that provides rehabilitation and support services to people who are blind and visually impaired. Call the number above or visit the website to find the office nearest you.

Canadian Mental Health Association, British Columbia Division

Telephone: (Vancouver) 604-688-3234 or 1-800-661-2121

Website: www.cmha-bc.org; Email: office@cmha-bc.org

Offers information on provincial mental health programs and provides support and assistance to families and caregivers. See its fact sheets on the website by clicking "Information and Resources."

Canadian Red Cross Society

Telephone: 250-382-2043 or 1-800-661-9055

Website: www.redcross.ca; Email: victoria@redcross.ca

Provides a number of home care services and equipment loans for eligible persons. Services vary by region; call your regional office to find specific services offered in your area.

Heart and Stroke Foundation of British Columbia & Yukon

Telephone: 604-736-4404

Website: www.heartandstroke.ca

Offers information and resources to help the understanding, prevention, and treatment of cardio/cerebrovascular disease. Call the above number or visit the website to find the office nearest you.

Multiple Sclerosis Society of Canada, British Columbia Division

Telephone: 604-689-3144 or 1-800-268-7582

Website: www.mssociety.ca/bc; Email: info.bc@mssociety.ca

Undertakes research into the cause and cure of multiple sclerosis and works to educate the public about the condition. Call the number above or visit the website to find the chapter nearest you.

Senior Information Centre

Telephone: 604-875-6381

Provides information on associations, resources, and organizations. It is for people who reside in the Lower Mainland only.

Seniors Medication Information Line (BC Smile)

Telephone: 604-822-1330 or 1-800-668-6233
Website: www.fvconnect.bc.ca/Chilliwack/health/bc-smile.htm;
Email:smileubc@unixg.ubc.ca

Operated by University of British Columbia licensed pharmacists, the line assists seniors and their caregivers with drug-related questions, especially those requiring extensive research (e.g., new medications, interactions, side effects, herbs, and vitamins).

SeniorsCan British Columbia Information

Website: www.crm.mb.ca/bc

The SeniorsCan Internet Program is a highly acclaimed guide for retirees and older adults to Canadian and global information and services. This is a very helpful website for British Columbia-based information.

Western Institute for the Deaf and Hard of Hearing

Telephone: 604-736-7391; (TTY/TDD) 604-736-2527
Website: www.widhh.com; Email: info@widhh.com

An information and service resource to people who are deaf and hard of hearing and to concerned individuals and agencies.

NURSING AND HOMEMAKING AGENCIES

For nursing and homemaking agencies in your area, please refer to NURSING AND HOMEMAKING AGENCIES in the Canada-wide listings.

HOME HEALTH CARE RETAILERS, HOME SAFETY AND ENVIRONMENT

There are a number of home health care retailers located throughout the province that can help you find the right products for your specific needs. To find a store near you, please refer to HOME HEALTH CARE RETAILERS, HOME SAFETY, AND ENVIRONMENT in the Canada-wide listings.

Canada Mortgage and Housing Corporation, British Columbia and Yukon Division

Telephone: 306-780-5880; (TTY) 1-888-841-4975

Website: www.cmhc.ca

See the Canada-wide listing under HOME HEALTH CARE RETAILERS, HOME SAFETY, AND ENVIRONMENT for services offered. Call the above number or visit the website to find the regional office nearest you.

FINANCIAL PLANNING/LEGAL

ABCs of Fraud Program

Telephone: 604-437-1940 or 1-866-437-1940

Website: www.bcceas.ca/fraud2.shtml; Email: ceas@telus.net

Provides group presentations in major centres across the country to educate seniors about fraud. The organization distributes complimentary support materials and provides referrals to additional resources. To book a presentation in Vancouver, call the 1-866 number above.

Community Legal Assistance Society

Telephone: 604-685-3425; (TTY) 604-685-8295

Website: www.orw.ca/source/legal/communit.htm; Email: clas@vancouver.net

Provides free legal assistance, in particular to those who are physically, mentally, or economically disadvantaged throughout B.C.

Legal Services Society

Telephone: 604-601-6000

Website: www.lss.bc.ca

Non-profit organization providing legal services and information to people who cannot afford a lawyer and legal education and information to the residents of B.C.

Office of the Public Guardian and Trustee

Telephone: 604-660-4444

Website: www.trustee.bc.ca; Email: mail@trustee.bc.ca

This office is responsible for protecting the financial rights of cognitively challenged people. The staff help individuals make decisions on personal care and medical treatment.

The office also advises family members on guardianship and on how to obtain the legal authority to make decisions on behalf of loved ones.

SUPPORT AGENCIES

Seniors Serving Seniors

Telephone: 250-382-4331

Website: www.seniorsservingseniors.bc.ca; Email: seniors@island.net

Seniors Serving Seniors was incorporated in 1981 as a non-profit society to promote the well-being of seniors in the Greater Victoria Area. It operates a set of programs designed to encourage and maintain social activation and community support networks. Services are free and provided by approximately 100 volunteers and one employee. Information and referrals are provided to all of the non-medical emergency resources available in the region, as well as personalized advice and expertise on many issues, including financial assistance, government services, housing, legal, personal support services, etc.

DRIVING CAPABILITY ASSESSMENT

In each province, the Ministry of Transportation makes the official decision on when a person must stop driving. The family physician is legally required to report any case in which someone's driving ability may be impaired due to the progression of age or any resulting condition. The physician must file his or her report with a medical review board, which may, based on research and interviews with key health care professionals, request a driving assessment to determine driving skills. Based on test results, a decision will be made on whether the individual will be allowed to continue to drive.

If you are concerned about your parents' ability to drive, you can request an independent assessment for one or both of them. Such assessments, which are provided by private companies for a fee, will help you determine your parents' safety while on the road.

B.C. Ministry of Transportation and Highways, Motor Vehicles Branch

Telephone: 250-978-8300

The government ministry that provides driver assessments to determine competence levels.

DriveAble Testing

Telephone: 604-321-2661 ext. 22617 or 1-877-433-1494

Website: www.driveable.com; Email: info@driveable.com

Driver assessment program for persons with possible cognitive impairment. Fee for service. Call the 1-877 number above for the testing centre nearest you.

CARING FOR YOURSELF

Caregivers Association of BC (CABC)

Telephone: 604-734-4812

Website: www.caregiverbc.ca; Email: cabc2000@vcn.bc.ca

CABC offers support, education, and information to unpaid family caregivers in B.C. Also provides training, manuals, reports, and other educational kits to help community leaders. Publishes *BC Caregiver News*.

Community Home Support Services Association

Telephone: 604-739-4300

Provides community-based, multi-level care services such as home support, total care for adults with developmental disabilities, and attendant care for persons with quadriplegia who are ventilator-dependent.

The Self-Help Resource Association of BC

Telephone: 604-733-6186

Website: www.vcn.bc.ca/shra; Email: shra@telus.net

This association was formed to meet the needs of the self-help community; it facilitates the development of self-help groups, peer support initiatives, networks, and resources. It also publishes the annual *Directory of Self-Help Support Groups in Greater Vancouver*.

Seniors' Foundation of British Columbia

Telephone: 604-685-4403

Website: www.seniorsbc.com

The Seniors' Foundation of British Columbia is committed to provide funding for projects that help seniors help themselves.

MANITOBA

GOVERNMENT

For a full list of programs and services offered by the federal government, please refer to FEDERAL GOVERNMENT in the Canada-wide listings.

The Manitoba Home Care Program is designed to help your parents live with dignity in their own home, for as long as safely possible. The local home care office should be your first point of access in Manitoba. There are a number of home care offices throughout the province. They are all are operated by one of the 11 regional health authorities. To locate your local home care office, check your local phone directory, call the Winnipeg Regional Health Authority at 204-926-7000, send an email to info@wrha.mb.ca, or visit the website at www.gov.mb.ca/health and click on "Regional Health Authorities" at the top of the page.

When you contact the local home care office, a health care professional will visit your parents and prepare a report, which will be forwarded to a panel of professionals who will review the application and determine the services and level of care required.

Manitoba Government Inquiry

Telephone: 1-800-626-4862 or 204-945-3744; (TDD) 204-945-4796
Email mgi@mb.ca

Provides direct communication between Manitobans and the provincial government. If you have a question but are not sure of the appropriate government department or agency to approach, this service will refer you to the correct office.

Manitoba Seniors and Healthy Aging Secretariat

Telephone: (Seniors' Information Line) 1-800-665-6565 or 204-945-6565
Website: www.gov.mb.ca/sd; Email: seniors@gov.mb.ca

A central point of contact for information and as a liaison with seniors, seniors' organizations, and government departments to ensure that government programs, policies, and legislation enhance the status of seniors.

Manitoba Health

Telephone: 204-945-3744 or 1-800-626-4862; (TDD) 204-945-4796
Website: www.gov.mb.ca/health; Email mgi@mb.ca

The website provides information on health services in the province and contact information for the regional health authorities, which can direct you to services in your area. If you prefer, call Manitoba Government Inquiry.

Pharmacare

Telephone: 1-800-297-8099 or 204-786-7141
Website: www.gov.mb.ca/health/pharmacare

Pharmacare is a drug benefit program for any Manitoban, regardless of age, whose income is seriously affected by high prescription drug costs.

The Seniors Abuse Help Line

Telephone: 1-888-896-7183 or 204-945-1884
Website: www.gov.mb.ca/sd/abuse

A confidential information service aimed at providing seniors, caregivers, and others with a one-stop information resource on elder abuse. There are useful publications available at the website.

LONG-TERM CARE FACILITIES

In Manitoba, there are two types of facilities that provide long-term care: supportive housing and personal care homes. Supportive housing provides light care; personal care homes provide a higher level of care.

An assessment is first conducted by a nurse to determine the person's needs. This assessment is then passed on to a central panel that decides what level of care is required. Based on this decision, a person may be referred to home support, respite care in the community, or a long-term care facility. For more information on assessments, contact your regional health authority or continuing care department at 204-788-6648.

GENERAL RESOURCES/SPECIAL NEEDS

Age and Opportunity

Telephone: 204-956-6440
Website: www.ageopportunity.mb.ca

A community service agency that offers a broad range of services to promote the health and wellness of older adults throughout Winnipeg. In addition, it operates a number of senior centres.

Alzheimer Society of Manitoba

Telephone: 204-943-6622 or 1-800-378-6699
Website: www.alzheimer.mb.ca; Email: alzmb@alzheimer.mb.ca

The central part of a volunteer-driven, three-tiered structure that links Alzheimer Canada with local Alzheimer groups in various Manitoba communities.

Arthritis Society, Manitoba Division

Telephone: 204-942-4892 or 1-800-321-1433;
(Western Manitoba) 204-729-9144
Website: www.arthritis.ca; Email: info@mb.arthritis.ca
or (Western Manitoba) hbernhardt@mb.arthritis.ca

A non-profit organization devoted to funding and promoting arthritis research, patient care, and public education.

Association for Community Living, Manitoba

Telephone: 204-789-9850
Website: www.aclmb.ca; Email: aclmb@mts.net

Advocates on behalf of people with intellectual disabilities to assist them in living a quality lifestyle through the development of community living programs.

Canadian Cancer Society, Manitoba Division

Winnipeg Office
Telephone: 204-774-7483 or 1-888-532-6982
Cancer Information Services: 1-888-939-3333
Website: www.mb.cancer.ca;
General email: resources@mb.cancer.ca or info.wpg@mb.cancer.ca
Brandon Office
Telephone: 204-571-2800 or 1-888-857-6658
Website: www.mb.cancer.ca;

General email: info.brandon@mb.cancer.ca

For information about cancer: info@cis.cancer.ca

Each divisional office provides various kinds of services; call to find out what is available.

Canadian Deafblind & Rubella Association, Manitoba Chapter

Telephone: 204-949-3730

Website: www.cdbra.ca; Email: intermb@mb.sympatico.ca

Provides intervention services to deaf-blind and rubella handicapped people throughout Manitoba.

Canadian Diabetes Association, Manitoba/Nunavut

Telephone: 204-925-3800 or 1-800-BANTING (1-800-226-8464)

Website: www.diabetes.ca; Email: mbinfo@diabetes.ca

A national, independent, self-financing organization that works to improve the quality of life of Canadians affected by diabetes by being the leading force in research, service, advocacy, and education. A very helpful website provides information to patients and professionals; patient information is available in English and Chinese. Call the number above for the local office nearest you.

Canadian Hard of Hearing Association, Manitoba Branch

Telephone: 204-975-2350

Website: www.chha.ca; Email: mbchha@mts.net

The association provides information and brochures on improving communication skills and helping people deal with hearing loss.

Canadian Mental Health Association, Manitoba Division

Telephone: 204-953-2350

Website: www.cmhamanitoba.mb.ca; Email: info@cmhamanitoba.mb.ca

Promotes mental health in Manitoba and advocates ensuring the best care, treatment, and rehabilitation for persons with emotional and mental problems. See the website or call the number above to find the branch nearest you.

Canadian National Institute for the Blind, Manitoba Division

Telephone: 204-774-5421

Website: www.cnib.ca/divisions/manitoba; Email: kris.owen@cnib.ca

A charitable, non-profit, voluntary agency that provides rehabilitation and support services to those who are blind and visually impaired. Call the number above or visit the website to find the district office near you.

Canadian Red Cross Society

Telephone: (Winnipeg/NE Manitoba) 204-982-7330;
(Western Manitoba) 204-729-4970
Website: www.redcross.ca

Provides a number of home care services and equipment loans for eligible persons. Services vary by region; call your regional office to find specific services offered in your area.

Contact Community Information

Telephone: 204-287-8827 or 1-866-266-4636
Website: www.contactmb.org; Email: projectvcw@mts.net

Refers Manitobans to social services and programs available through health, educational, cultural, and recreational resources in the province.

Heart and Stroke Foundation of Manitoba

Telephone: 204- 949-2000 or 1-888-473-4636
Website: www.heartandstroke.ca

Provides free literature on a wide range of topics such as controlling stress and cholesterol, managing high blood pressure, and smoking cessation. Call the above number or visit the website to find the office nearest you.

Meals on Wheels of Winnipeg, Inc.

Telephone: 204-956-7711
Website: www3.mb.sympatico.ca/~meals;
Email: meals@mealsonwheelswpg.ca

Provides nutritious meals delivered by volunteers to those in the community unable to prepare or otherwise obtain them.

Multiple Sclerosis Society of Canada, Manitoba Division

Telephone: 204-943-9595 or 1-800-268-7582

Website: www.mssociety.ca/manitoba; Email: info.manitoba@mssociety.ca

Undertakes research into the cause and cure of multiple sclerosis and works to educate the public about the condition. Call the number above or visit the website to find the chapter nearest you.

SeniorsCan Manitoba Information

Website: www.crm.mb.ca/mb

The SeniorsCan Internet Program is a highly acclaimed guide for retirees and older adults to Manitoban, Canadian, and global information and services. This is a very useful website for Manitoba-specific information.

NURSING AND HOMEMAKING AGENCIES

For nursing and homemaking agencies in your area, please refer to NURSING AND HOMEMAKING AGENCIES in the Canada-wide listings.

HOME HEALTH CARE RETAILERS, HOME SAFETY AND ENVIRONMENT

There are a number of home health care retailers located throughout the province that can help you find the right products for your specific needs. To find a store near you, please refer HOME HEALTH CARE RETAILERS, HOME SAFETY, AND ENVIRONMENT in the Canada-wide listings.

Canada Mortgage and Housing Corporation, Prairie, Nunavut and Northwest Territories Division

Telephone: 204-983-5600; (TTY) 1-888-841-4975

Website: www.cmhc.ca

See the Canada-wide listing under HOME HEALTH CARE RETAILERS, HOME SAFETY, AND ENVIRONMENT for services offered. Call the above number or visit the website to find the office nearest you.

FINANCIAL PLANNING/LEGAL

ABCs of Fraud Program

Telephone: 604-437-1940 or 1-866-437-1940

Website: www.bcceas.ca/fraud2.shtml; Email: ceas@telus.net

Offers group presentations in major centres across the country to educate seniors about fraud, distributes complimentary support materials, and provides referrals to additional resources. To book a presentation in Winnipeg, call the 1-866 number above.

Legal Aid Manitoba

Telephone: 204-985-8500 or 1-800-261-2960

Website: www.legalaid.mb.ca

Legal Aid Manitoba can fully or partially fund a lawyer to represent a person or group in a lawsuit. Individuals must complete an application and be found eligible. Legal Aid also offers informal drop-in services for simpler questions.

Office of the Vulnerable Persons' Commissioner

Telephone: 204-945-5039 or 1-800-757-9857

Website: www.gov.mb.ca/fs/pwd/vpo.html; Email: spd@gov.mb.ca

This office protects the rights of adults living with a mental disability, helps individuals make decisions on personal care and medical treatment, and advises family members on guardianship and on how to obtain the legal authority to make decisions on behalf of loved ones.

DRIVING CAPABILITY ASSESSMENT

In each province, the Ministry of Transportation makes the official decision on when a person must stop driving. The family physician is legally required to report any case in which someone's driving ability may be impaired due to the progression of age or any resulting condition. The physician must file his or her report with a medical review board, which may, based on research and interviews with key health care professionals, request a driving assessment to determine driving skills. Based on test results, a decision will be made on whether the individual will be allowed to continue to drive.

If you are concerned about your parents' ability to drive, you can request an independent assessment for one or both of them. Such assessments, which are provided by private companies for a fee, will help you determine your parents' safety while on the road. Contact the department listed below for more information.

Manitoba Highways and Government Services, Medical Review Section

Telephone: 204-945-7386

This department provides driver assessments to determine driving competence.

Creative Retirement Manitoba

Telephone: 204-949-2565

Website: www.crm.mb.ca/crm; Email: denesiuk@crm.mb.ca

Offers a number of programs and services for seniors including Fully Alive and the 55 Alive/Mature Driving course.

NEW BRUNSWICK

GOVERNMENT

For a full list of programs and services offered by the federal government, please refer to FEDERAL GOVERNMENT in the Canada-wide listings.

In New Brunswick, home and community health care services are offered through the Department of Family and Community Service regional offices. The Department will conduct an assessment and financial evaluation to determine the level of care required. Based upon this evaluation, you will then be referred to the correct services your parents require. Whenever possible, individuals are expected to contribute financially to their care. To locate a Family and Community Service office near you, call 506-453-2001.

The fourth edition (2002) of the *Seniors' Guide to Services and Programs* is available in English or French on the Internet at www.gnb.ca/0017/Seniors/SeniorsGuide-e.pdf or by calling 506-453-2082.

Providing Care and Assistance to Older Family Members is another helpful publication available in online format at www.gnb.ca/0017/Seniors/hints-e.asp.

Family and Community Social Services
Telephone: 506-453-2001
Website: www.gnb.ca/0017

This department offers long-term and in-home support services based on assessments and eligibility (depending on the level of needs of the individual). It also provides case management and referrals to various service providers. The website has a section of practical hints for caregivers.

Prescription Drug Program
Telephone: 506-453-3983 or 1-800-332-3692
Website: www.gnb.ca/0212/seniors-e.asp

Provides prescription drug benefits to eligible residents of New Brunswick. The program is targeted to those with a demonstrated medical and financial need.

Service New Brunswick

Telephone: 506-684-7901 or 1-888-762-8600
Telephone link to government services.

LONG-TERM CARE FACILITIES

In New Brunswick, there are two types of long-term care facilities: special care homes and nursing homes. Special care homes are for people who can care for themselves; nursing homes provide a higher level of support and are for people who require 24-hour care.

Admission to either is based on a referral from a family physician or by contacting the Department of Family and Community Services (see GOVERNMENT above) to obtain information and start the process. Requires an assessment conducted by a public health nurse or social worker to determine the necessary level of care and funding required and any other needs. Admission is based on the assessment.

GENERAL RESOURCES/SPECIAL NEEDS

Alzheimer Society of New Brunswick

Telephone: 506-459-4280;
Family Information and Referral Line) 1-800-664-8411
Website: www.alzheimer.nb.ca; Email: info@alzheimernb.ca

This organization is the central part of a volunteer-driven, three-tiered structure that links Alzheimer Canada with local Alzheimer groups in various New Brunswick communities. Check the website or call the 1-800 number to find the office and services nearest you.

Arthritis Society, New Brunswick Division

Telephone: 506-452-7191 or 1-800-321-1433
Website: www.arthritis.ca; Email: info@nb.arthritis.ca

The Arthritis Society is a non-profit organization devoted to funding and promoting arthritis research, patient care, and public education.

The Blue Cross Seniors' Health Program

Telephone: 1-800-565-0065

Provides access to the New Brunswick Drug Program for those residents of the province who are not otherwise eligible.

Canadian Cancer Society, New Brunswick Division

Telephone: 506-634-6272

Cancer Information Service: 1-888-939-3333

Website: www.nb.cancer.ca; General email: ccsnb@nb.cancer.ca

For information about cancer: info@cis.cancer.ca

Each divisional office provides various kinds of services; call to find out what is available.

Canadian Deafblind & Rubella Association, New Brunswick/PEI Chapter

Telephone: 506-452-1544

Website: www.deafblind.nb.ca; Email: cdbra@nbnet.ca

Provides intervention services to deaf-blind and rubella handicapped people throughout New Brunswick and Prince Edward Island.

Canadian Diabetes Association, New Brunswick

Telephone: 506-452-9009 or 1-800-884-4232

Website: www.diabetes.ca; Email: nbinfo@diabetes.ca

A national, independent, self-financing organization that works to improve the quality of life of Canadians affected by diabetes by being the leading force in research, service, advocacy, and education. A very helpful website provides information to patients and professionals; patient information is available in English and Chinese. Call the number above for the local office nearest you.

Canadian Hard of Hearing Association, New Brunswick Branch

Telephone: 506-472-6941

Website: www.chha.ca; Email: mary.currie@brunnet.net

Provides information and brochures on improving communication skills and helping people deal with hearing loss.

Canadian Mental Health Association, New Brunswick Division

Telephone: 506-455-5231

Website: www.cmhanb.ca; Email: cmhanb@nbnet.nb.ca

Promotes mental health in New Brunswick and advocates ensuring the best care, treatment, and rehabilitation for persons with emotional and mental problems. For branches throughout the province, visit the website or call the number above.

Canadian National Institute for the Blind, New Brunswick Division.

Telephone: 506-458-0060

Website: www.cnib.ca/divisions/nbeng

A charitable, non-profit, voluntary agency that provides rehabilitation and support services to people who are blind and visually impaired. Call the number above or visit the website to find the district office nearest you.

Canadian Red Cross Society

Telephone: 506-674-6200

Offers a variety of services to seniors throughout the province including homecare, meals on wheels, equipment loan programs, and a unique home partner program.

Canadian Rehabilitation Council for the Disabled, New Brunswick Branch

Telephone: 506-458-8739

Helps people of all ages who may have physical disabilities achieve maximum rehabilitation.

Chimo Crisis Line

Telephone: 1-800-667-5005

A toll-free, 24-hour, province-wide telephone helpline for people who are experiencing a crisis.

Greater Saint John Seniors' Directory

Telephone: 506-633-4636

Website: www.town.grandbay-westfield.nb.ca/rec/senserv.htm

A useful directory of a wide range of services for seniors in the Saint John area, including listings for counselling and support, elder abuse, housing, recreation, and respite services.

Heart and Stroke Foundation of New Brunswick

Telephone: 506-634-1620 or 1-800-663-3600

Website: www.heartandstroke.ca; Email: heart.strokemail@nb.aibn.com

Provides free literature on a wide range of topics such as controlling stress and cholesterol, managing high blood pressure, and smoking cessation.

New Brunswick Senior Citizens' Federation

Telephone: 1-800-453-4333 or 506-857-8242

Website: www.sjfn.nb.ca/community_hall/N/newb8242.html

Strives for awareness of the human community and its environment by exploring issues relevant to seniors.

Multiple Sclerosis Society of Canada, Atlantic Division

Telephone: 902-468-8230

Website: www.mssociety.ca/atlantic; Email: info.atlantic@mssociety.ca

Undertakes research into the cause and cure of multiple sclerosis and works to educate the public about the condition.

New Brunswick Association for Community Living

Telephone: 506-453-4400 or 1-866-622-2548

Website: www.nbacl.nb.ca; Email: nbacl@nbnet.ca

Works with people who have intellectual disabilities and their families to build inclusive communities where those with intellectual disabilities can live, learn, work, and actively participate in their communities as valued and contributing members.

SeniorsCan New Brunswick Information

Website: www.crm.mb.ca/nb

The SeniorsCan Internet Program is a highly acclaimed guide for retirees and older adults to Canadian and global information and services. This website contains very useful New Brunswick specific information.

Tele-Care

Telephone: 1-800-244-8353

Website: www.gnb.ca/0217/Tele-Care-e.asp

A bilingual, province-wide, 24-hour service for help with non-emergency medical problems.

NURSING AND HOMEMAKING AGENCIES

For nursing and homemaking agencies in your area, please refer to NURSING AND HOMEMAKING AGENCIES in the Canada-wide listings.

HOME HEALTH CARE RETAILERS, HOME SAFETY AND ENVIRONMENT

There are a number of home health care retailers located throughout the province that can help you find the right products for your specific needs. To find a store near you, please refer to HOME HEALTH CARE RETAILERS, HOME SAFETY, AND ENVIRONMENT in the Canada-wide listings.

Canada Mortgage and Housing Corporation, Atlantic Provinces Division

Telephone: 506-452-3050

Website: www.cmhc.ca

See the Canada-wide listing under HOME HEALTH CARE RETAILERS, HOME SAFETY, AND ENVIRONMENT for services offered. Call the above number or visit the website to find the regional office nearest you.

VOLUNTEER AGENCIES

Senior Goodwill Ambassador Program

Telephone: 506-457-6811

Website: www.gnb.ca/0017/Seniors/goodwill-e.asp

Part of a government project initiated in order to promote New Brunswick at home and abroad. Use the skills of volunteer retirees 65 years of age and older to make presentations to schools, community colleges, service clubs, and businesses on the positive aspects of New Brunswick.

FINANCIAL PLANNING/LEGAL

ABCs of Fraud Program

Telephone: 1-866-437-1940

Website: www.bcceas.ca/fraud2.shtml; Email: ceas@telus.net

Provides group presentations in major centres across the country to educate seniors about fraud, distributes complimentary support materials, and provides referrals to additional resources. To book a presentation in Saint John, call the 1-866 number above.

DRIVING CAPABILITY ASSESSMENT

In each province, the Ministry of Transportation makes the official decision on when a person must stop driving. The family physician is legally required to report any case in which driving ability may be impaired due to the progression of age or any resulting condition. The physician must file his or her report with a medical review board, which may, based on research and interviews with key health care professionals, request a driving assessment to determine driving skills. Based on test results, a decision will be made on whether the individual will be allowed to continue to drive.

If you are concerned about your parents' ability to drive, you can request an independent assessment for one or both of them. Such assessments, which are provided by private companies for a fee, will help you determine your parents' safety while on the road. Contact the department below for more information.

New Brunswick Department of Transportation

Telephone: 506-453-3939

This department provides driver assessments to determine driving competence.

Vehicle Retrofitting and Accessible Vehicle Program

Telephone: 506-453-5818

Website: www.gnb.ca/0113/Policy/vretro/veh-retrofit-e.asp;
Email: claudette.mcallister@gnb.ca

This program is designed to provide assistance for retrofitting vehicles with eligible accessibility features.

NEWFOUNDLAND AND LABRADOR

GOVERNMENT

For a full list of programs and services offered by the federal government, please refer to FEDERAL GOVERNMENT in the Canada-wide listings.

There are six health and community services boards in Newfoundland that look after home care and other related services for aging parents with special needs. Once you contact your local office, a health care professional will visit your parent and conduct an assessment. This assessment will help determine your parent's needs and the level of care that he or she may require. Call the Department of Health and Community Services at 709-729-4984 or email healthinfo@gov.nl.ca to locate the office nearest to you.

LONG-TERM CARE FACILITIES

There are a number of facilities throughout the province that provide varying levels of care. Your local community health board has a complete list. Your care coordinator will be able to direct you to the proper facility based on the level of care that your parent requires.

GENERAL RESOURCES/SPECIAL NEEDS

Alzheimer Society of Newfoundland and Labrador

Telephone: 709-576-0608 or 1-877-776-0608
Website: www.alzheimer.ca; Email: sharing@avalon.nf.ca

The Alzheimer Society provides educational and support programs to improve awareness and to assist families and individuals coping with the disease, as well as information on resources, phone support, guest speakers, support groups, community resources, and a number of innovative programs throughout the province. Check the website or call the toll-free number for details on the chapter nearest you.

Arthritis Society, Newfoundland and Labrador Division

Telephone: 709-579-8190 or 1-800-321-1433

Wesite: www.arthritis.ca/nl; Email: info@nl.arthritis.ca

A non-profit organization devoted to funding and promoting arthritis research, patient care, and public education.

Canadian Cancer Society, Newfoundland & Labrador Division

Telephone: 709-753-6520 or 1-888-753-6520

Cancer Information Service: 1-888-939-3333

Website: www.cancer.ca; General email: ccs@nl.cancer.ca

For information about cancer: info@cis.cancer.ca

Each divisional office provides various kinds of services; call to find out what is available.

Canadian Diabetes Association, Newfoundland & Labrador

Telephone: 709-754-0953 or 1-800-BANTING (226-8464)

Website: www.diabetes.ca; Email: carolann.smith@diabetes.ca

An national, independent, self-financing organization that works to improve the quality of life of Canadians affected by diabetes by being the leading force in research, service, advocacy, and education.

Canadian Hard of Hearing Association, Newfoundland Branch

Telephone: 709-753-3224

Website: www.chha-nc.nf.ca; Email: chhanc@nfld.net

Provides information and brochures on improving communication skills and helping people deal with hearing loss.

Canadian Mental Health Association, Newfoundland Division

Telephone: 709-753-8550 or 1-866-509-3937

Website: www.cmhanl.ca; Email: office@cmhanl.ca

This divisional office works to promote understanding of mental health and mental illness through education, advocacy, and community development.

Canadian National Institute for the Blind, Newfoundland and Labrador Division

Telephone: 709-754-1180 or 1-800-334-2642

Website: www.cnib.ca/divisions/nfllrd

The Canadian National Institute for the Blind offer numerous resources including counselling and referral, orientation and mobility training, sight enhancement, and technical aids. Call the above toll-free number or visit the website to find the office nearest you.

Canadian Red Cross Society

Telephone: 709-758-8400

Website: www.redcross.ca

Provides a number of home care services and equipment loans for eligible persons. Services vary by region; call your regional office to find specific services offered in your area.

Heart and Stroke Foundation of Newfoundland and Labrador

Telephone: 709-753-8521

Website: www.heartandstroke.ca

Provides free literature on a wide range of topics such as controlling stress and cholesterol, managing high blood pressure, and smoking cessation.

SeniorsCan Newfoundland & Labrador Information

Website: www.crm.mb.ca/nf

The SeniorsCan Internet Program is a highly acclaimed guide for retirees and older adults to Canadian and global information and services. This website offers helpful Newfoundland and Labrdor specific information.

Seniors' Resource Centre

Telephone: 709-737-2333 or 1-800-563-5599

Website: www.infornet.st-johns.ca/providers/seniors;

Email: seniorsresource@ng.aibn.com

The centre offers a number of programs for caregivers, including a free newsletter and a Friday friendship club, as well as friendly visiting and other community services. Operates a toll-free line for unpaid caregivers at 1-888-571-2273.

NURSING AND HOMEMAKING AGENCIES

For nursing and homemaking agencies in your area, please refer to NURSING AND HOMEMAKING AGENCIES in the Canada-wide listings.

HOME HEALTH CARE RETAILERS, HOME SAFETY AND ENVIRONMENT

There are a number of home health care retailers located throughout the province that can help you find the right products for your specific needs. To find a store near you, please refer to HOME HEALTH CARE RETAILERS, HOME SAFETY, AND ENVIRONMENT in the Canada-wide listings.

Canada Mortgage and Housing Corporation, Atlantic Provinces Division

Telephone: 709-772-4400
Website: www.cmhc.ca

See the Canada-wide listing under HOME HEALTH CARE RETAILERS, HOME SAFETY, AND ENVIRONMENT for services offered. Call the above number or visit the website for the office nearest you.

FINANCIAL PLANNING/LEGAL

ABCs of Fraud Program

Telephone: 1-866-437-1940
Website: www.bcceas.ca/fraud2.shtml; Email: ceas@telus.net

Provides group presentations in major centres across the country to educate seniors about fraud. It distributes complimentary support materials and provides referrals to additional resources. To book a presentation in St. John's, call the 1-866 number above.

Office of the Public Guardian and Trustee

Telephone: 709-729-0850
Email: karenelawlor@hotmail.com

This office is responsible for protecting the financial rights of cognitively challenged people. It helps individuals make decisions on personal care and medical treatment. The office also advises family members on guardianship and on how to obtain the legal authority to make decisions on behalf of loved ones.

DRIVING CAPABILITY ASSESSMENT

In each province, the Ministry of Transportation makes the official decision on when a person must stop driving. The family physician is legally required to report any case in which someone's driving ability may be impaired due to the progression of age or any resulting condition. The physician must file his or her report with a medical review board, which may, based on research and interviews with key health care professionals, request a driving assessment to determine driving skills. Based on test results, a decision will be made on whether the individual will be allowed to continue to drive.

If you are concerned about your parents' ability to drive, you can request an independent assessment for one or both of them. Such assessments, which are provided by private companies for a fee, will help you determine your parents' safety while on the road. Contact the department below for more information.

Newfoundland Department of Works, Services and Transportation

Telephone: 709-729-2300

This department provides driver assessments to determine driving competence.

NORTHWEST TERRITORIES

GOVERNMENT

For a full list of programs and services offered by the federal government, please refer to FEDERAL GOVERNMENT in the Canada-wide listings.

The Department of Health and Social Services provides programs and services related to senior care, such as Extended Health Benefit Seniors Program, HomeCare, Long Term Care, Seniors Home Heating Subsidy Program, and many others. Call 867-873-7925, visit the website (www.hlthss.gov.nt.ca), or email dianne_mercredi@gov.nt.ca for details. Visit the Seniors Policies and Programs Database at www.sppd.gc.ca/ and click on "Northwest Territories" for a comprehensive listing in one place.

GENERAL RESOURCES

Alzheimer Society of Alberta and Northwest Territories

Telehpone: 403-250-1303
Email: yellowknife@alzheimer.ab.ca

The Alzheimer Society provides educational and support programs to improve awareness and to assist families and individuals coping with the disease. The resource centre is open to the public and can provide referrals to support groups in your local area and mail information. Provides services to Yellowknife and Northwest Territory residents.

Canadian Cancer Society, Alberta & NWT Division

Northwest Territories Section: 867-920-4428
Cancer Information Service: 1-888-939-3333
Website: www.cancer.ca; Email: arleney@cancer.ab.ca
For information about cancer: info@cis.cancer.ca

There are a variety of services provided, including support groups. Call the office number above to find out what is available near you.

Canadian Diabetes Association, Alberta & NWT Regions

Northern Alberta and NWT: 780-423-1232 or 1-800-563-0032

Website: www.diabetes.ca; Email: freda.badry@diabetes.ca

A national, independent, self-financing organization that works to improve the quality of life of Canadians affected by diabetes by being the leading force in research, service, advocacy, and education. A very helpful website provides information to patients and professionals; patient information is available in English and Chinese. Call the number above for the local office nearest you.

Canadian Mental Health Association, Northwest Territories Division

Telephone: 867-873-3190; (Inuvik) 867-979-4148; (Baffin) 867-979-4151

Promotes mental health and advocates ensuring the best care, treatment, and rehabilitation for persons with emotional and mental problems.

Canadian National Institute for the Blind, Alberta-Northwest Territories-Nunavut Division

Telephone: (Yellowknife) 867-873-2647

The Canadian National Institute for the Blind offers numerous resources, including counselling and referral, orientation and mobility training, sight enhancement, and technical aids.

Heart and Stroke Foundation of Alberta, NWT and Nunavut

Telephone: 1-888-473-4636

Provides free literature on a wide range of topics such as controlling stress and cholesterol, managing high blood pressure, and smoking cessation.

Northwest Territories Seniors Information Line

Telephone: 1-800-661-0878

Email: seniors@tamarack.nt.ca

A one-stop information line to provide information on seniors programs and services, pensions and benefits, and other issues that relate to seniors.

NURSING AND HOMEMAKING AGENCIES

For nursing and homemaking agencies in your area, please contact the Home Care Section of the Department of Health and Social Services at 867-920-8746.

HOME HEALTH CARE RETAILERS, HOME SAFETY AND ENVIRONMENT

A social/intake worker at the territorial home care program will be able to find you the home health care products you require.

Canada Mortgage and Housing Corporation, Prairie, Nunavut and Northwest Territories Division

Telephone: 867-873-2637

Website: www.cmhc.ca

See the Canada-wide listing under HOME HEALTH CARE RETAILERS, HOME SAFETY, AND ENVIRONMENT for services offered. Call the above number or visit the website to find the office nearest you.

FINANCIAL PLANNING/LEGAL

Legal Services Board, Law Line

Telephone: (Yellowknife only) 920-2360 or 1-867-873-3130

This board is responsible for ensuring that all eligible people in the Northwest Territories receive legal services. The board follows prescribed guidelines for determining if a person is eligible and oversees the operations of legal aid clinics situated in every administrative region of the N.W.T. If you require further information about legal aid, the legal system, or if you have a specific legal problem, you can call the Law Line and speak to a lawyer for free and in confidence.

Office of the Public Guardian and Trustee

Telephone: 867-873-7464 or 1-866-535-0423

Website: www.justice.gov.nt.ca; Email: larry_pontus@gov.nt.ca

This office is responsible for protecting the financial rights of cognitively challenged people. It helps individuals make decisions on personal care and medical treatment. The office also advises family members on guardianship and on how to obtain the legal authority to make decisions on behalf of parents.

DRIVING CAPABILITY ASSESSMENT

In each province and territory, the Ministry of Transportation makes the official decision on when a person must stop driving. Your family physician is legally required to report any case in which someone's driving ability may be impaired due to the progression of age or any resulting condition. The physician must file his or her report with a medical review board, which may, based on research and interviews with key health care professionals, request a driving assessment to determine driving skills. Based on test results, a decision will be made on whether the individual will be allowed to continue to drive.

If you are concerned about your parents' ability to drive, you can request an independent assessment for one or both of them. Such assessments, which are provided by private companies for a fee, will help you determine your parents' safety while on the road. For a private assessment, please see DriveAble in the DRIVING CAPABILITY ASSESSMENT section for Alberta.

Northwest Territories Transportation
Telephone: 867-873-7406

This department provides driver assessments to determine driving competence.

NOVA SCOTIA

GOVERNMENT

For a full list of programs and services offered by the federal government, please refer to FEDERAL GOVERNMENT in the Canada-wide listings.

Public Enquiries Officers respond to telephone enquiries about all provincial government services, programs, and initiatives. The service offers a province-wide toll-free telephone line at 1-800-670-4357; the local number is 902-424-5200.

Health care service delivery is provided through one of nine district health authorities. Each is responsible for delivering all care services to people in its particular region. In addition, the Nova Scotia Department of Health has established a toll-free number that will direct you to the closest facility. Call the Nova Scotia Department of Health at 902-424-5815 or 1-800-387-6665. You can send an email to dohweb@gov.ns.ca or visit the website at www.gov.ns.ca/health for a list of programs and services and access to the websites of the district health authorities.

Nova Scotia Department of Health: Continuing Care Branch

Telephone: 1-800-225-7225; (Out of province) 1-902-424-4288
Website: www.gov.ns.ca/health/ccs

This office serves people who need ongoing care outside of hospital, either on a long-term or short-term basis. Its services include home care, long-term care, and protection for vulnerable adults.

Nova Scotia Department of Health: Long-Term Care

Telephone: 902-424-4476

This department of the Continuing Care Branch provides information and referrals to long-term care facilities, such as nursing and retirement homes. An assessment is first conducted to determine the individual's level of care.

Senior Citizens' Secretariat and Seniors Information Line

Telephone: (Halifax/Dartmouth) 902-424-0065; 1-800-670-0065

Website: www.gov.ns.ca/scs

A comprehensive listing of provincial government services for seniors. The publication *Programs for Seniors* is updated annually and is available online or as a booklet. The website offers some very useful links to information on topics such as health, safety, legal matters, and retirement/leisure.

LONG-TERM CARE FACILITIES

There are a number of facilities throughout the province that provide varying levels of care. Your local district health authority has a complete list. Your care coordinator will be able to direct you to the proper facility based on the level of care that your parent requires. For more information about home care and long-term care services, call 1-800-225-7225.

GENERAL RESOURCES/SPECIAL NEEDS

Alzheimer Society of Nova Scotia

Telephone: 902-422-7961 or 1-800-611-6345

Website: www.alzheimer.ns.ca; Email: info@alzheimer.ns.ca

The Alzheimer Society provides educational and support programs to improve awareness and to assist families and individuals coping with the disease, information on resources, phone support, guest speakers, support groups, community resources, and a number of innovative programs throughout the province. One program is an eight-week course administered through the QE II Hospital, which deals with overall caregiving issues for people in the early stages of dementia.

Arthritis Society, Nova Scotia Division

Telephone: 902-429-7025 or 1-800-321-1433

Website: www.arthritis.ca; Email: info@ns.arthritis.ca

A non-profit organization devoted to funding and promoting arthritis research, patient care, and public education.

Canadian Cancer Society, Nova Scotia Division

Telephone: 902-423-6183 or 1-800-639-0222

Cancer Information Services: 1-888-939-3333

Website: www.cancer.ca; General email: ccs.ns@ns.cancer.ca

For information about cancer: info@cis.cancer.ca

Each divisional office provides various kinds of services; call to find out what is available.

Canadian Diabetes Association, Nova Scotia

Telephone: 902-453-4CDA (4232) or 1-800-326-7712;

(Cape Breton) 902-564-6461

Website: www.diabetes.ca; Email: arelene.parsons@diabetes.ca

A national, independent, self-financing organization that works to improve the quality of life of Canadians affected by diabetes by being the leading force in research, service, advocacy, and education.

Canadian Mental Health Association

Telephone: 902-466-6600

Website: www.cmhans.org; Email: cmhans@allstream.net

Promotes mental health in Nova Scotia and advocates ensuring the best care, treatment, and rehabilitation for persons with emotional and mental problems. For branches throughout the province, visit the website or call the number above.

Canadian National Institute for the Blind, Nova Scotia-Prince Edward Island Division

Telephone: 902-453-1480 or 1-800-565-5147

Website: www.cnib.ca/divisions/nspei

The Canadian National Institute for the Blind offers numerous resources including counselling and referral, orientation and mobility training, sight enhancement, and technical aids. Call the above number or visit the website to find the office nearest you.

Canadian Red Cross Society

Telephone: 902-423-3680

Website: www.redcross.ca

Provides a number of home care services and equipment loans for eligible persons. Services vary by region; call your regional office to find specific services offered in your area.

Caregiver Resource Library

Telephone: 902-457-6561

Website: www.msvu.ca/nsca/Library.asp; Email: nsca@msvu.ca

Located at the Nova Scotia Centre on Aging at Mount Saint Vincent University, the library offers more than 1,000 books, videos, and other resources related to caregiving and aging available to lend free of charge. You can download a copy of its catalogue on the website. You will need Adobe Acrobat to do this, which you can obtain free at www.adobe.com/products/acrobat/readstep2.html.

Continuing Care Association of Nova Scotia

Telephone: 902-453-2977

Website: www.nsnet.org/ccans; Email: ccans@ns.aliantzinc.ca

CCANS is a not-for-profit organization representing some 50 facilities and service providers that offer residential care or various support services for the elderly with special needs.

Heart and Stroke Foundation of Nova Scotia

Telephone: 902-423-7530

Website: www.heartandstroke.ca

Provides free literature on a wide range of topics such as controlling stress and cholesterol, managing high blood pressure, and smoking cessation.

Late-Deafened Adult Support Group

Telephone: 902-434-1673; (TTY) 902-477-2396

Provides emotional support and resources to residents in the Halifax area.

Multiple Sclerosis Society of Canada, Atlantic Division

Telephone: 902-468-8230 or 1-800-268-7582

Website: www.mssociety.ca/atlantic; Email: info.atlantic@mssociety.ca

Undertakes research into the cause and cure of multiple sclerosis and works to educate the public about the condition.

Nova Scotia Association of Health Organizations

Telephone: 902-832-8500
Website: www.nsaho.ns.ca

Represents more than 100 organizations, including nine district health authorities, 50 continuing care providers, and home care and home support agencies.

SeniorsCan Nova Scotia Information

Website: www.crm.mb.ca/ns

The SeniorsCan Internet Program is a highly acclaimed guide for retirees and older adults to Canadian and global information and services. This website provides very useful Nova Scotia specific information.

Society of Deaf and Hard of Hearing Nova Scotians

Telephone: 902-422-7130
Website: www.sdhhns.org; Email: sdhhns@ns.sympatico.ca

Assists adult deaf, deafened, and hard of hearing Nova Scotians to gain access to existing public, private, and community services.

NURSING AND HOMEMAKING AGENCIES

For nursing and homemaking agencies in your area, please refer to NURSING AND HOMEMAKING AGENCIES in the Canada-wide listings.

HOME HEALTH CARE RETAILERS, HOME SAFETY AND ENVIRONMENT

There are a number of home health care retailers located throughout the province that can help you find the right products for your specific needs. To find a store near you, please refer HOME HEALTH CARE RETAILERS, HOME SAFETY, AND ENVIRONMENT in the Canada-wide listings.

Canada Mortgage and Housing Corporation, Atlantic Provinces Division

Telephone: 902-426-3530
Website: www.cmhc.ca

See the Canada-wide listing under HOME HEALTH CARE RETAILERS, HOME SAFETY, AND ENVIRONMENT for services offered. Call the above number or visit the website for the office nearest you.

FINANCIAL PLANNING/LEGAL

Legal Information Society of Nova Scotia

Telephone: 902-454-2198
Legal Information Line/Lawyer Referral Service: 902-455-3135 or
1-800-665-9779
Website: www.legalinfo.org

Provides information and resources about wills, family, power of attorney, and other legal matters.

Nova Scotia Legal Aid

Telephone: 902-9 420-3471
Website: www.gov.ns.ca/just/legad.htm

There are 13 regional offices and 3 sub-offices in the province. Legal aid may be provided to people on social assistance or in an equivalent financial position in certain areas of family and criminal law. Check the phone directory or call the number above for the Nova Scotia Legal Aid office nearest you.

Public Trustee of Nova Scotia

Telephone: 902-424-7760
Website: www.gov.ns.ca/just/pubtrustee.htm

This office is responsible for protecting the financial rights of cognitively challenged people. It helps individuals make decisions on personal care and medical treatment and advises family members on guardianship and on how to obtain the legal authority to make decisions on behalf of loved ones. The Public Trustee also manages the estates of people who need services of a trustee, guardian, or attorney not readily available in the private sector.

VOLUNTEER AGENCIES

Good Neighbours

Telephone: 902-424-0065 or1-800-670-0065

Encourages people to reach out and help one another and to create caring, sharing, and friendly communities.

Family Caregivers Association of Nova Scotia

Telephone: 902-421-7390 or 1-877-488-7390

Website: www.caregiversns.org; Email: fcgans@caregiversns.org

This non-profit organization offers information and practical support for all caregivers, whether family, friends, or neighbours. It provides newsletter and other resources and has a strong network with other caregiving groups throughout the province.

Volunteer Resource Centre - Sydney

Telephone: 902-562-1245

Website: www.newdawn.ca; Email: vrc@newdawn.ca

Coordinates and administers Meals on Wheels, Each One Teach One, a friendly visiting service, transportation, and snow-shovelling. It is a non-profit organization and a member of the United Way of Cape Breton.

DRIVING CAPABILITY ASSESSMENT

In each province, the Ministry of Transportation makes the official decision on when a person must stop driving. The family physician is legally required to report any cases in which driving ability may be impaired due to the progression of age or any resulting condition. The physician must then file his or her report with a medical review board, which may, based on research and interviews with key health care professionals, request a driving assessment to determine driving skills. Based on test results, a decision will be made on whether the individual will be allowed to continue to drive.

0If you are concerned about your parents' ability to drive, you can request an independent assessment for each or both of them. Such assessments, which are provided by private companies for a fee, will help you determine your parents' safety while on the road. Contact the department below for more information.

Registry of Motor Vehicles: Medical Section

Telephone: 902-424-5732

This department provides driver assessments to determine driving competence. A voluntary assessment will be charged a fee; an assessment that is requested by a physician or the ministry is free of charge.

DriveAble Testing

Telephone: 902-423-2605 or 1-877-433-1494
Website: www.driveable.com; Email: info@driveable.com

Driver assessment program available in Halifax for people with possible cognitive impairment. Fee for service.

Nova Scotia Safety Council 55 Alive

Telephone: 902-454-9621

A national mature driver refresher course. The course, free to those 65 years and over, consists of six hours of classroom instruction only, commonly offered over two mornings. There are no tests and no negative effects on the licence.

GOVERNMENT

For a full list of programs and services offered by the federal government, please refer to FEDERAL GOVERNMENT in the Canada-wide listings.

Nunavut Ministry of Health
Telephone: 867-979-7601

This department provides information on provincial health services and departments related to home care and caring for aging parents.

GENERAL RESOURCES

Canadian National Institute for the Blind, Alberta-Northwest Territories-Nunavut
Telephone: (Calgary office) 403-266-8831; 1-800-367-2642

The Canadian National Institute for the Blind offers numerous resources including counselling and referral, orientation and mobility training, sight enhancement, and technical aids.

Heart and Stroke Foundation of Alberta, NWT and Nunavut
Telephone: 1-888-473-4636

Provides free literature on a wide range of topics such as controlling stress and cholesterol, managing high blood pressure, and smoking cessation.

NURSING AND HOMEMAKING AGENCIES

For nursing and homemaking agencies in your area, please contact the Nunavut Ministry of Health at 867-979-7601.

HOME HEALTH CARE RETAILERS, HOME SAFETY AND ENVIRONMENT

A social/intake worker at the Territorial Ministry of Health will be able to find you the home health care products you require. Call 867-979-7601.

Canada Mortgage and Housing Corporation, Prairie, Nunavut and Northwest Territories Division

Telephone: (Calgary office) 403-515-3000; (TTY) 1-888-841-4975

Website: www.cmhc.ca

See the Canada-wide listing under HOME HEALTH CARE RETAILERS, HOME SAFETY, AND ENVIRONMENT for services offered. Call the above number or visit the website to find the office nearest you.

FINANCIAL PLANNING/LEGAL

Office of the Public Guardian and Trustee

Telephone: 867-975-5700

This office is responsible for protecting the financial rights of cognitively challenged people. It helps individuals make decisions on personal care and medical treatment. The office also advises family members on guardianship and on how to obtain the legal authority to make decisions on behalf of parents.

DRIVING CAPABILITY ASSESSMENT

In each province and territory, the Ministry of Transportation makes the official decision on when a person must stop driving. Your family physician is legally required to report any case in which someone's driving ability may be impaired due to the progression of age or any resulting condition. The physician must file his or her report with a medical review board, which may, based on research and interviews with key health care professionals, request a driving assessment to determine driving skills. Based on test results, a decision will be made on whether the individual will be allowed to continue to drive.

If you are concerned about your parents' ability to drive, you can request an independent assessment for one or both of them. Such assessments, which are provided by private companies for a fee, will help determine your parents' safety while on the road. For an assessment, please see DriveAble in the DRIVING CAPABILITY ASSESSMENT section for Ontario.

Motor Vehicles Department

Telephone: 867-873-7419

This department provides driver assessments to determine driving competence.

ONTARIO

GOVERNMENT

For a full list of programs and services offered by the federal government, please refer to FEDERAL GOVERNMENT in the Canada-wide listings.

Forty-three Community Care Access Centres (CCAC) located throughout the province serve as the entry point to the Ontario community health care system. The local CCAC will conduct an assessment and direct you and your parents to the resources and services that are required.

In addition, you may be able to access private services (such as a nursing or home-making agency) from independent associations and organizations through the local CCAC. The centre also will provide you with information on other important caregiving resources such as support groups, crisis lines, related health care associations, and long-term care facilities.

To locate the Community Care Access Centre in your area, call 1-800-268-1154 (Ontario Ministry of Health) or the CCAC head office at 416-750-1720 or visit its website at www.oaccac.on.ca. Call 1-877-234-4343 to receive a free copy of its publication *What's Right for Me* guide to care options.

Assistive Devices and Home Oxygen Programs
Telephone: 416-327-4282; 1-800-268-6021; (TTY) 1-800-387-5559
Website: www.health.gov.on.ca/english/public/program/adp/adp_mn.html
These programs offer financial assistance for those who have a prescribed need for home care products such as wheelchairs, scooters, walkers, etc. It also provides home oxygen services.

Information and Referral Service for Vulnerable Adults and Seniors
Telephone: 416-482-4359; 1-800-665-9092; (TTY) 1-800-387-5559
Free telephone referral service that provides information to persons with disabilities including Alzheimer's or dementia.

Ministry of Health and Long Term Care:
Health Information Centre

Telephone: 1-800-268-1154

Website: www.health.gov.on.ca

This provincial office is responsible for health care delivery within Ontario. The ministry provides referrals to provincial services (including Community Care Access Centres) that offer specific assistance for different kinds of needs. At its website, click on the menu selection "Home, Community, & Residential Care Services for Seniors" to go to the web page that discusses care options.

Ontario Seniors' Secretariat

Telephone: 416-326-7076; 1-888-910-1999; 1-800-387-5559

Website: www.gov.on.ca/mczcr/seniors

Provides access a variety of information of interest to seniors, their families, and those who work with seniors.

Telehealth Ontario

Telephone: 1-866-797-0000

Call to speak to a nurse about medical or health-related issues.

LONG-TERM CARE FACILITIES

There are a number of long-term care facilities throughout the province that provide varying levels of care. Your local Community Care Access Centre has a complete list of local facilities. Your care coordinator will be able to direct you to the proper facility based on the level of care that your loved one requires. In addition, there are numerous retirement homes that provide light, supportive care. The association listed below will help you find the proper facility.

GENERAL RESOURCES/SPECIAL NEEDS

Ontario Residential Care Association

Telephone: 905-403-0500 or 1-800-361-7254

Website: www.orca-homes.com; Email: info@orca-homes.com

A voluntary, self-regulating organization representing over 250 retirement homes caring for more than 17,000 residents. ORCA operates a consumer information service and publishes a free consumer directory of member facilities. Go to the website or call the above number for a free copy of its publication *The Care Guide*, a directory of retirement residences in Ontario.

The Care Guide

Telephone: 416-287-2273 or 1-800-311-2273
Website: www.thecareguide.com

Operated by CARE Planning Partners Inc., this site provides information on seniors' housing and care services. The site features provider search tools, community bulletin boards, and an online assessment tool. A print copy of its directory is available online or by calling the above number.

GENERAL RESOURCES/SPECIAL NEEDS

Alzheimer Society of Ontario

Telephone: 416-967-5900
Website: www.alzheimerontario.org

The Alzheimer Society provides educational and support programs to improve awareness and to assist families and individuals coping with the disease; also provides support groups, education sessions, and guest speakers. Check the website or get in touch with the provincial office for details on the office nearest you.

The Arthritis Society, Ontario Division

Telephone: (Toronto) 416-979-7228; 1-800-321-1433
Website: www.arthritis.ca; Email: info@on.arthritis.ca

This is a non-profit organization devoted to funding and promoting arthritis research, patient care, and public education.

Canadian Cancer Society, Ontario Division

Telephone: 416-488-5400 or 1-800-268-8874
Cancer Information Services: 1-888-939-3333
Website: www.ontario.cancer.ca
For information about cancer: info@cis.cancer.ca

Each divisional office provides various kinds of services; call to find out what is available. Visit the website or call the above number to find the branch nearest you.

Canadian Deafblind & Rubella Association

Telephone: 519-759-0520 or 1-877-760-7439

Website: www.cdbra.ca; Email: cathy@cdbraontario.ca

Provides intervention services to deaf-blind and rubella handicapped people throughout Ontario.

Canadian Diabetes Association, Ontario

Telephone: 1-800-BANTING (226-8464)

Website: www.diabetes.ca

A national, independent, self-financing organization that works to improve the quality of life of Canadians affected by diabetes by being the leading force in research, service, advocacy, and education. A very helpful website provides information to patients and professionals; patient information is available in English and Chinese. Call the 1-800 number above to locate the branch nearest you.

Canadian Hard of Hearing Association, Ontario Branch

Telephone: 416-338-1695

Website: www.chha.ca; Email: ralexander@toronto.ca

The association provides information and brochures on improving communication skills and helping people deal with hearing loss. Call the above number or visit the website to find the branch nearest you.

Canadian Mental Health Association

Telephone: 416-977-5580

Website: www.ontario.cmha.ca; Email: info@ontario.cmha.ca

Promotes mental health in Ontario and advocates ensuring the best care, treatment, and rehabilitation for people with emotional and mental problems. See the website or call the number above to find the branch nearest you.

Canadian National Institute for the Blind, Ontario Division

Telephone: 416-413-9480; (TTY) 416-480-8645

Website: www.cnib.ca/division/ontario

The Canadian National Institute for the Blind offers numerous resources including counselling and referral, orientation and mobility training, sight enhancement, and technical aids. Call the number above or visit the website to find the office nearest you.

Canadian Red Cross Society

Telephone: 905-890-1000
Website: www.redcross.ca

Provides a number of home care services and equipment loans for eligible persons. Services vary by region; call your regional office to find specific services offered in your area.

Consumer Health Information Service (CHIS)

Telephone: 416-393-7056 or 1-800-667-1999
Website: www.tpl.toronto.on.ca/uni_chi_index.jsp

CHIS provides names of relevant associations and resources as a starting point to help consumers make more informed decisions about their own health care. CHIS mails out custom packages of helpful information for consumers who live outside the Greater Toronto Area.

Heart and Stroke Foundation of Ontario

Telephone: 416-489-7111
Website: www.heartandstroke.ca

Provides free literature on a wide range of topics such as controlling stress and cholesterol, managing high blood pressure, and smoking cessation. Call the above number or visit the website to find the provincial office nearest you.

Services for Seniors

Telephone: 416-481-4579
Website: www.services4seniors.ca; Email: info@services4seniors.ca

Provides drop-in senior companions for various services, including driving, overnight and 24-hour live-in support, and home cleaning. Fee for service.

SeniorsCan Ontario Information

Website: www.crm.mb.ca/on

The SeniorsCan Internet Program is a highly acclaimed guide for retirees and older adults to Canadian and global information and services. This is a very useful website for Ontario-specific information.

NURSING AND HOMEMAKING AGENCIES

For nursing and homemaking agencies in your area, please refer to NURSING AND HOMEMAKING AGENCIES in the Canada-wide listings.

Ontario Home Health Care Providers Association

Website: www.homecareontario.ca

An organization of home health and social care providers. The website has very useful links to current information about home health care in Ontario.

St. Elizabeth Health Care

Telephone: 905-940-9655
Website: www.saintelizabeth.com;
Email: communications@saintelizabeth.com

A non-profit nursing agency with a full range of nursing and homemaking services available throughout Ontario, and consulting services to other agencies across Canada.

HOME HEALTH CARE RETAILERS, HOME SAFETY AND ENVIRONMENT

There are a number of home health care stores located throughout the province that can help you find the right products for your specific needs. To find a store near you, please refer to HOME HEALTH CARE RETAILERS, HOME SAFETY, AND ENVIRONMENT in the Canada-wide listings.

Canada Mortgage and Housing Corporation, Ontario Division

Telephone: 416-221-2642; (TTY) 1-800-309-3388
Website: www.cmhc.ca

See the Canada-wide listing under HOME HEALTH CARE RETAILERS, HOME SAFETY, AND ENVIRONMENT for services offered. Call the above number or visit the website for the office nearest you.

FINANCIAL PLANNING/LEGAL

ABCs of Fraud Program

Telephone: 604-437-1940 or 1-866-437-1940

Website: www.bcceas.ca/fraud2.shtml; Email: ceas@telus.net

Provides group presentations in major centres across the country to educate seniors about fraud, distributes complimentary support materials, and provides referrals to additional resources. To book a presentation in Toronto, call the 1-866 number above.

Advocacy Centre for the Elderly

Telephone: 416-598-2656

Website: www.advocacycentreelderly.org

A legal clinic for low-income, 60+ seniors in the Greater Toronto Area. ACE offers one-on-one legal advice and provides updates on new legislation relevant to the rights of seniors. Most of the ACE services are provided free of charge.

Legal Aid Ontario

Telephone: 416-979-1446 or 1-800-668-8258

Website: www.legalaid.on.ca; Email: info@lao.on.ca

Legal aid is available to lower-income people for a variety of legal issues. Eligibility is based on financial need and the type of case. The applicant may pay nothing or a portion of the costs of the legal aid, depending on his or her financial situation. Once approved, a legal aid certificate entitles a person to retain the lawyer of his or her choice. The lawyer is then reimbursed by Legal Aid Ontario.

Legal Line

Telephone: 416-929-6011 ext. 725

Website: www.legalline.ca; Email info@legalline.ca

Provides free legal information to residents of Ontario through the phone and Internet. The service will provide Ontario residents with sufficient legal information to know when the assistance of a lawyer is advisable and direct them to the Ontario Bar and other appropriate resources for further assistance.

Office of the Public Guardian and Trustee

**For assistance with treatment decisions,
call 416-314-2788 or 1-800-387-2127.
To report a situation involving an adult whom you believe to be mentally
incapable and suffering or at risk of suffering or serious harm,
contact 416-327-6348 or 1-800-366-0335.**

This office is responsible for protecting the financial rights of cognitively challenged people. It helps individuals make decisions on personal care and medical treatment. The office also advises family members on guardianship and on how to obtain the legal authority to make decisions on behalf of loved ones.

DRIVING CAPABILITY ASSESSMENT

In each province, the Ministry of Transportation makes the official decision on when a person must stop driving. The family physician is legally required to report any case in which someone's driving ability may be impaired due to age or any resulting condition. The physician must file his or her report with a medical review board, which may, based on research and interviews with key health care professionals, request a driving assessment to determine driving skills. Based on test results, a decision will be made on whether the individual will be allowed to continue to drive.

If you are concerned about your parents' ability to drive, you can request an independent assessment for one or both of them. Such assessments, which are provided by private companies for a fee, will help you determine your parents' safety while on the road.

Ontario Ministry of Transportation

Telephone: 416-235-2999 or 1-800-387-3445

This department provides driver assessments to determine driving competency.

DriveAble Testing

**Telephone: 416-498-6429 or 1-877-433-1494
Website: www.driveable.com; Email: info@driveable.com**

Driver assessment program for persons with possible cognitive impairment. Fee for service. Call the 1-877 number above to find the testing centre nearest you.

CARING FOR YOURSELF

Self Help Resource Centre

Telephone: 416-487-4355 or 1-888-283-8806

Website: www.selfhelp.on.ca; Email: shrc@selfhelp.on.ca

Provides listings of self-help groups across Ontario for family, friends, and caregivers looking after aging parents, and many other self-help categories.

Ontario Community Support Association

Telephone: 416-256-3010 1-800-267-6272

Website: www.ocsa.on.ca

A good resource to connect to some 360 agencies across Ontario providing a host of services, including meals on wheels, many of which will be relevant to caregivers, including referrals to organizations that offer therapeutic counselling and relief from caregiving duties.

PRINCE EDWARD ISLAND

GOVERNMENT

For a full list of programs and services offered by the federal government, please refer to FEDERAL GOVERNMENT in the Canada-wide listings.

In P.E.I., contacting your local regional health board is your first step in finding the home care resources you need. Each region has a Home Care Office that offers a variety of services. Upon contacting the local office, a health care professional will visit your home and conduct an assessment. This assessment will help the professional to determine your parent's needs and the level of care that he or she requires. To locate the Home Care Office nearest you, check your local phone directory or visit the comprehensive provincial website at www.gov.pe.ca/seniors.

Another very good resource is the province-wide Health Information Resource Centre; call 1-800-241-6970, email hirc@gov.pe.ca , or visit www.gov.pe.ca/hirc. At this website, you can access the Health & Wellness Resource Centre, a searchable, online database of medical journals and articles on health issues in plain language that is available to Island residents only; you will need to enter the first half of your postal code to access the database. The helpful Directory of Self-Help Groups and Community Resources is available by calling 902-566-3034 or 1-800-682-1648.

PEI Department of Health and Social Services

Telephone: 902-368-4900
Website: www.gov.pe.ca/hss

This department provides information on provincial health services and departments related to home care.

LONG-TERM CARE FACILITIES

Nursing care is accessed by contacting a placement officer in one of the five health regions on P.E.I. There are a number of facilities throughout the province that provide varying levels of care. Your local Home Care Office has a complete list. Your care coordinator will be able to direct you to the proper facility based on the level of care that your loved one requires.

GENERAL RESOURCES/SPECIAL NEEDS

Alzheimer Society of PEI

Telephone: 902-628-2257
Email: society@alzpei.ca

The Alzheimer Society provides educational and support programs to improve awareness and to assist families and individuals coping with the disease, as well as information on books, resources, phone support, guest speakers, support groups, community resources, and a number of innovative programs throughout the province.

Arthritis Society, PEI Division

Telephone: 902-628-2288 or 1-800-321-1433
Website: www.arthritis.ca; Email: info@pe.arthritis.ca

A non-profit organization devoted to funding and promoting arthritis research, patient care, and public education.

Canadian Cancer Society, PEI Division

Telephone: 902-566-4007 or 1-866-566-4007
Cancer Information Services: 1-888-939-3333
Website: www.pei.cancer.ca; Email: info@pei.cancer.ca

Each divisional office provides various kinds of services; call to find out what is available.

Canadian Diabetes Association, Prince Edward Island

Telephone: 902-894-3005 or 1-800-BANTING (226-8464)
Website: www.diabetes.ca; Email: berry@diabetes.ca

A national, independent, self-financing organization that works to improve the quality of life of Canadians affected by diabetes by being the leading force in research, service, advocacy, and education.

Canadian Mental Health Association, Prince Edward Island Division

Telephone: 902-566-3034

Website: www.cmha.pe.ca; Email: division@cmha.pe.ca

Promotes mental health in P.E.I. and advocates ensuring the best care, treatment, and rehabilitation for persons with emotional and mental problems. For branches throughout the province, see the website or call the number above.

Canadian National Institute for the Blind, Nova Scotia-Prince Edward Island Division

Telephone: (Charlottetown) 902-566-2580

Website: www.cnib.ca/divisions/nspei

A charitable, non-profit, voluntary agency that provides rehabilitation and support services to people who are blind and visually impaired.

Canadian Red Cross Society

Telephone: 902-628-6262

Website: www.redcross.ca

Provides a number of home care services and equipment loans for eligible persons. Services vary by region; call your regional office to find specific services offered in your area.

Heart and Stroke Foundation of PEI

Telephone: 902-892-7441

Website: www.heartandstroke.ca

Provides free literature on a wide range of topics such as controlling stress and cholesterol, managing high blood pressure, and smoking cessation.

Island Help Line

Telephone: 1-800-218-2885

The Island Help Line is a 24-hour, free, confidential service providing information, support, and crisis counselling on family matters, child abuse, alcohol and drugs, parenting, and suicide.

Multiple Sclerosis Society of Canada, Atlantic Division

Telephone: 902-468-8230 or 1-800-268-7582

Website: www.mssociety.ca/atlantic; Email: info.atlantic@mssociety.ca

Undertakes research into the cause and cure of multiple sclerosis and works to educate the public about the condition.

PEI Senior Citizens' Federation

Telephone: 902-628-8388

Website: www.crm.mb.ca/pe/peiscf.html

The purpose of the federation is to further the interests and promote the happiness and welfare of senior citizens and pensioners in Prince Edward Island in every way possible. This chapter has its own newspaper, holds workshops across the Island, and advocates for seniors.

Prince Edward Island Association for the Hearing Impaired

Telephone: 902-892-6585

Provides services and information for the hearing impaired in P.E.I.

SeniorsCan Prince Edward Island Information

Website: www.crm.mb.ca/pe

The SeniorsCan Internet Program is a highly acclaimed guide for retirees and older adults to Canadian and global information and services. This is a very useful website for P.E.I. information.

NURSING AND HOMEMAKING AGENCIES

For nursing and homemaking agencies in your area, please refer to NURSING AND HOMEMAKING AGENCIES in the Canada-wide listings.

HOME HEALTH CARE RETAILERS, HOME SAFETY AND ENVIRONMENT

There are a number of home health care retailers located throughout the province that can help you find the right products for your specific needs. To find a store near you, please refer to HOME HEALTH CARE RETAILERS, HOME SAFETY, AND ENVIRONMENT in the Canada-wide listings.

Canada Mortgage and Housing Corporation, Atlantic Provinces Division

Telephone: 902-566-7079

Website: www.cmhc.ca

See the Canada-wide listing under HOME HEALTH CARE RETAILERS, HOME SAFETY, AND ENVIRONMENT for services offered. Call the above number or visit the website to find the office nearest you.

FINANCIAL PLANNING/LEGAL

Office of the Public Guardian and Trustee

Telephone: 902-368-4933

This office is responsible for protecting the financial rights of cognitively challenged people. It helps individuals make decisions on personal care and medical treatment. The office also advises family members on guardianship and on how to obtain the legal authority to make decisions on behalf of loved ones.

VOLUNTEER AGENCIES

Seniors Info Line

Telephone: 902-368-7538

Provides access to information about services that support seniors in their wish to remain in their own homes as long as possible.

Charlottetown Meals on Wheels Inc.

Telephone: 902-569-7700

Provides nutritious meals and social contact to those who cannot obtain adequate nutrition on their own. Run by volunteers.

DRIVING CAPABILITY ASSESSMENT

In each province, the Ministry of Transportation makes the official decision on when a person must stop driving. The family physician is legally required to report any case in which someone's driving ability may be impaired due to the progression of age or any resulting condition. The physician must file his or her report with a medical review board, which may based on research and interviews with key health care professionals, request a driving assessment to determine driving skills. Based on test results, a decision will be made on whether the individual will be allowed to continue to drive.

If you are concerned about your parents' ability to drive, you can request an independent assessment for one or both of them. Such assessments, which are provided by private companies for a fee, will help you determine your parents' safety while on the road. Contact the department below for more information.

PEI Transportation and Public Works
Telephone: 902-368-5100

This department provides driver assessments to determine driving competence.

PEI Safety Council
Telephone: 902-894-7500 or 1-800-618-4697

Offers the 55 Alive seniors driving course.

GOVERNMENT

For a full list of programs and services offered by the federal government, please refer to FEDERAL GOVERNMENT in the Canada-wide listings.

The Quebec government has a very centralized approach to providing information about its services. Communication-Québec is its principal information arm, providing comprehensive lists and descriptions of services available. Call 1-800-363-1363 or visit the website at www.gouv.qc.ca/Accueil/LeSaviezVous/LangueGrappes_en.html and download the PDF file with extensive listings. Centres Locaux de Service Communitaires (CLSCs) are located throughout the province of Quebec and are your first contact for finding the health care services you need. Each CLSC provides a number of services, including nursing care, home care and domestic help, and referrals to outside agencies. You can find the closest CLSC by calling the Association des CLSC at 514-931-1448.

LONG-TERM CARE FACILITIES

There are a number of facilities throughout the province that provide varying levels of care. Your local CLSC has a complete list. Your care coordinator will be able to direct you to the proper facility based on the level of care that parent requires.

GENERAL RESOURCES/SPECIAL NEEDS

Fédération québécoise des sociétés alzheimer
(Federation of Quebec Alzheimer Societies)

Telephone: (Montreal) 514-369-7891; 1-888-636-6473
Website: www.alzheimerquebec.ca; Email: info-fqsa@alzheimerquebec.ca

The Alzheimer Society provides educational and support programs to improve awareness and to assist families and individuals coping with the disease. This provincial association will refer callers to regional offices of the Alzheimer's society that, in turn, will provide a variety of services for caregivers of persons with dementia or

Alzheimer's. For example, the Alzheimer Society of Montreal offers support groups and provides informational brochures, pamphlets, etc. Check the website or call the federation office to find the office nearest you.

Canadian Arthritis Society

Telephone: (Montreal) 514-846-8840; 1-800-321-1433

A non-profit organization devoted to funding and promoting arthritis research, patient care, and public education. Contact the Montreal office to find the office and services nearest you.

Canadian Cancer Society, Quebec Division

Telephone: 514-255-5151
Cancer Information Service: 1-888-939-3333
Website: www.quebec.cancer.ca;
General email: webmestre@quebec.cancer.ca
For information about cancer: info@cis.cancer.ca

Each divisional office provides various kinds of services; call to find out what is available.

Canadian Hard of Hearing Association, Quebec Branch

Telephone: 613-526-1584

This association provides information and brochures on improving communication skills and helping people deal with hearing loss.

Association cannadienne pour la santé mentale, Division du Québec (Canadian Mental Health Association, Quebec Division)

Telephone: 514-849-3291
Website: www.acsm.qc.ca; Email: acsm@cam.org

Promotes mental health in Quebec and advocates ensuring the best care, treatment, and rehabilitation for persons with emotional and mental problems. For branches throughout the province, visit the website or call the number above.

Canadian Red Cross Society

Telephone: 514-362-2930
Website: www.redcross.ca

Provides a number of home care services and equipment loans for eligible persons. Services vary by region; call your regional office to find specific services offered in your area.

Diabète Québec

Telephone: 514-254-3422 ext. 233 or 1-800-361-3504 ext. 233
Website: www.diabete.qc.ca; Email: info@diabete.qc.ca

Diabète Québec provides services, information, education, and advocacy for those with diabetes. The website is available in English and French.

Heart and Stroke Foundation of Quebec

Telephone: 514-871-1551
Website: www.heartandstroke.ca

The foundation provides information on a wide range of topics such as controlling stress and cholesterol, managing high blood pressure, and smoking cessation. It offers a very informative website. Call the above number or visit the website to find the office nearest you.

Héma Québec

Telephone: 514-832-5000 or 1-888-666-4362
Website: www.hema-quebec.qc.ca; Email: info@hema-quebec.qc.ca

The Quebec equivalent of the Canadian Blood Services.

L'institut national canadien pour les aveugles Division du Québec (Canadian National Institute for the Blind, Quebec Division)

Telephone: 514-934-4622 or 1-800-465-4622
Website: (in French only) www.cnib.ca/divisions/quebec;
Email: susan.vida.@inca.ca

The Canadian National Institute for the Blind offers numerous resources, including counselling and referral, orientation and mobility training, sight enhancement, and technical aids.

SeniorsCan Quebec Information

Website: www.crm.mb.ca/qc

The SeniorCan Internet Program is a highly acclaimed guide for retirees and older adults to Canadian and global information and services. This website contains very useful Quebec information.

Nursing and Homemaking Agencies

For nursing and homemaking agencies in your area, please refer to Nursing and Homemaking Agencies in the Canada-wide listings.

Home Health Care Retailers, Home Safety and Environment

There are a number of home health care retailers located throughout the province that can help you find the right products for your specific needs. To find a store near you, please refer to Home Health Care Retailers, Home Safety, and Environment in the Canada-wide listings.

Canada Mortgage and Housing Corporation, Quebec Division

Telephone: 514-283-2222
Website: www.cmhc.ca

See the Canada-wide listing under Home Health Care Retailers, Home Safety, and Environment for services offered. Call the above number or visit the website for the office nearest you.

Financial Planning/Legal

Curateur public du Quebec (Public Trustee)

Telephone: 514-873-4074 or 1-800-363-9020
Website: www.curateur.gouv.qc.ca/cura;
Email: information@curateur.gouv.qc.ca

This office is responsible for protecting the financial rights of cognitively challenged people. It helps individuals make decisions on personal care and medical treatment, offers power of attorney kits and wills, and helps search for heirs and next-of-kin. The office also advises family members on guardianship and on how to obtain the legal authority to make decisions on behalf of loved ones.

Commission des services juridiques (Legal Aid)

Telephone: 514-873-3562
Website: www.csj.qc.ca; Email: info@csj.qc.ca

Legal Aid offers economically disadvantaged people access to the courts, the professional services of an attorney or a notary, and the information they need regarding their rights and obligations. Eligibility for legal aid is based on several factors, including the applicant's family obligations, income, property, and liquid assets. People eligible are entitled to the services of a legal aid lawyer. They also are entitled to a lawyer in private practice if he or she accepts; however, not all services are covered.

DRIVING CAPABILITY ASSESSMENT

In each province, the Ministry of Transportation makes the official decision on when a person must stop driving. The family physician is legally required to report any case in which driving ability may be impaired due to the progression of age or any resulting condition. The physician must then file his or her report with a medical review board, which may, based on research and interviews with key health care professionals, request a driving assessment to determine driving skills. Based on test results, a decision will be made on whether the individual is allowed to continue to drive.

If you are concerned about your parents' ability to drive, you can request an independent assessment for one or both of them. Such assessments, which are provided by private companies for a fee, will help you determine your parents' safety while on the road.

Ministère des Transports du Québec

Telephone: 1-888-355-0511

Website: www.mtq.gouv.qc.ca

This department provides driver assessments to determine driving competence.

DriveAble Testing

Telephone: 514-733-1414 or 1-877-433-1494

Website: www.driveable.com; Email: info@driveable.com

Driver assessment program for persons with possible cognitive impairment. Fee for service. Call the 1-877 number above to find the testing centre nearest you.

SASKATCHEWAN

GOVERNMENT

For a full list of programs and services offered by the federal government, please refer to FEDERAL GOVERNMENT in the Canada-wide listings.

In Saskatchewan, 32 district health boards and one health authority in the north are responsible for all health care within the province. They are your first step to finding the services you need in your area. The health boards and health authority hire their own staff and do not contract work out to independent companies. Phone the Saskatchewan Health and Social Services Department of Community Care at 306-787-1501 for the district health board nearest you. Long-term care facilities are also referred through this system.

Information is also available through the Saskatchewan Association of Health Organizations: SAHO Regina: 306-347-5500; SAHO Saskatoon: 306-374-3480, www.saho.org.

Housing Territory Operations Offices
Telephone: (Northern Saskatchewan) 1-800-667-9656;
(Southern Saskatchewan) 1-800-814-8688
Website:
www.dcre.gov.sk.ca/housing/programs/seniors_families_disabile.html#seniors;
Email: communication@dcre.gov.sk.ca

Saskatchewan has a number of housing programs to assist seniors including: Affordable Housing Rentals (seniors rentals), Home Adaptations for Seniors' Independence (HASI), Saskatchewan Assisted Living Services (SALS), and Social Housing Rental Program — Seniors Rentals, and the Rent Supplement Program. Call the above number or visit the website for more information.

Saskatchewan Aids to Independent Living
Telephone: 306-787-7121
Website: www.health.gov.sk.ca/ps_sail.html

Equipment is available on a loan basis if requisitioned by a designated health professional.

Saskatchewan Health Community Care Branch

Telephone: 306-787-7126
Website: www.health.gov.sk.ca/ph_br_community_care.html;
Email: ccbweb@health.gov.sk.ca

Helps develop and support community programs such as home care, safe driving, and special care (nursing) homes.

LONG-TERM CARE FACILITIES

There are a number of facilities throughout the province that provide varying levels of care. Your local district health board has a complete list. Your care coordinator will be able to direct you to the proper facility based on the level of care that your loved one requires.

GENERAL RESOURCES/SPECIAL NEEDS

Alzheimer Society of Saskatchewan

Telephone: 306-949-4141 or 1-800-263-3367
Website: www.alzheimer.sk.ca; Email: info@alzheimer.sk.ca

Provides educational and support programs to improve awareness and to assist families and individuals coping with the disease; also offers support groups, education sessions, and a care-at-home service department that trains nurses, health care aids, etc., for at-home work. All at-home services are fee based and are reviewed on a case-by-case basis to determine eligibility for financial aid. Check the website or call the provincial office for details on the office and services nearest you.

Arthritis Society, Saskatchewan Division

Telephone: 1-800-321-1433; 306-352-3312; (Saskatoon) 306-244-9922
Website: www.arthritis.ca; Email: info@sk.arthritis.ca

A non-profit organization devoted to funding and promoting arthritis research, patient care, and public education.

Canadian Cancer Society, Saskatchewan Division

Telephone: 306-522-7347 or 1-877-977-HOPE (4673)
Cancer information services: 1-888-939-3333
Website: www.sk.cancer.ca; Email: ccssk@sk.cancer.ca

Each divisional office provides various kinds of services; call to find out what is available.

Canadian Deafblind & Rubella Association, Saskatchewan Chapter

Telephone: 306-374-0022

Website: www.cdbra.ca; Email: lorraine.cdbra@sk.shaw.ca

Provides intervention services to deaf-blind and rubella handicapped people throughout Saskatchewan.

Canadian Diabetes Association, Saskatchewan

Telephone: (North) 306-933-1238 or 1-800-996-4446;
(South) 306-584-8445 or 1-800-297-7488

Website: www.diabetes.ca; Email: (North) vaidyanathan@diabetes.ca or
(South) jordan.ball@diabetes.ca

A national, independent, self-financing organization that works to improve the quality of life of Canadians affected by diabetes by being the leading force in research, service, advocacy, and education. A very helpful website provides information to patients and professionals; patient information is available in English and Chinese. Call the number above for the local office nearest you.

Canadian National Institute for the Blind, Saskatchewan Division

Telephone: 306-525-2571

Website: www.cnib.ca/divisions/saskatchewan

The CNIB offers numerous resources, including counselling and referral, orientation and mobility training, sight enhancement, and technical aids. Call the number above or visit the website to find the district office nearest you.

Canadian Mental Health Association, Saskatchewan Division

Telephone: 306-525-5601 or 1-800-461-5483

Website: www.cmhask.com; Email: cmhask@accesscomm.ca

Promotes mental health in Saskatchewan and advocates ensuring the best care, treatment, and rehabilitation for people with emotional and mental problems. Check the website or call the toll-free number above to find the branch office nearest you.

Canadian Red Cross Society

Telephone: (Southern Saskatchewan) 306-721-1600; (Prince Albert) 306-765-2600; (Saskatoon) 306-668-0720

Website: www.redcross.ca

Provides a number of home care services and equipment loans for eligible persons. Services vary by region; call your regional office to find specific services offered in your area.

Heart and Stroke Foundation of Saskatchewan

Telephone: 306-244-2124

Website: www.heartandstroke.ca

Provides free literature on a wide range of topics such as controlling stress and cholesterol, managing high blood pressure, and smoking cessation. Call the above number or visit the website to find the one nearest you.

Multiple Sclerosis Society of Canada, Saskatchewan Division

Telephone: 306-522-5600 or 1-800-268-7582

Website: www.mssociety.ca/sask; Email: info.sask@mssociety.ca

Undertakes research into the cause and cure of multiple sclerosis and works to educate the public about the condition

Saskatchewan Association for Community Living

Telephone: 306-955-3344

Website: www.sacl.org; Email: sacl@sacl.org

Helps aging individuals with an intellectual disability. Support services and counselling are based on need. Call the above number or send an email to find the branch nearest you.

Saskatchewan Deaf and Hard of Hearing Services Inc.

Telephone: (Regina) 306-352-3323 or 1-800-565-3323; (Saskatoon) 306-665-6575 or 1-800-667-6575

Website: www.sdhhs.com; Email: (Regina) regina@sdhhs.com or (Saskatoon) saskatoon@sdhhs.com

This non-profit organization serves deaf, hard of hearing, and late-deafened persons with a variety of support services. These include communication services, social work, and hearing aid battery sales.

SeniorsCan Saskatchewan Information

Website: www.crm.mb.ca/sk

The SeniorsCan Internet Program is a highly acclaimed guide for retirees and older adults to Canadian and global information and services. This very useful website contains Saskatchewan specific information.

NURSING AND HOMEMAKING AGENCIES

For nursing and homemaking agencies in your area, please refer to NURSING AND HOMEMAKING AGENCIES in the Canada-wide listings.

HOME HEALTH CARE RETAILERS, HOME SAFETY AND ENVIRONMENT

There are a number of home health care retailers located throughout the province that can help you find the right products for your specific needs. To find a store near you, please refer HOME HEALTH CARE RETAILERS, HOME SAFETY, AND ENVIRONMENT in the Canada-wide listings.

Canada Mortgage and Housing Corporation, Prairie, Nunavut and Northwest Territories Division

Telephone: 306-780-5880; (TTY) 1-888-841-4975

Website: www.cmhc.ca

See the Canada-wide listing under HOME HEALTH CARE RETAILERS, HOME SAFETY, AND ENVIRONMENT for services offered. Call the above number or visit the website to find the office nearest you.

FINANCIAL PLANNING/LEGAL

Office of the Public Guardian and Trustee

Telephone: 306-787-5424
Website: www.saskjustice.gov.sk.ca/PublicTrustee;
Email: pgt@justice.gov.sd.ca

This office is responsible for protecting the property of people who do not have the capacity to manage their own financial affairs. It helps individuals make decisions on personal care and medical treatment and advises family members on guardianship and on how to obtain the legal authority to make decisions on behalf of loved ones.

Saskatchewan Legal Aid Commission

Telephone: 306-933-5300 or 1-800-667-376
Email: central@legalaid.gov.sd.ca

Provides legal services to people who can't afford a lawyer. Call or email to find the office nearest you.

DRIVING CAPABILITY ASSESSMENT

In each province, the Ministry of Transportation makes the official decision on when a person must stop driving. The family physician is legally required to report any case in which someone's driving ability may be impaired due to the progression of age or any resulting condition. The physician must then file his or her report with a medical review board, which may, based on research and interviews with key health care professionals, request a driving assessment to determine driving skills. Based on test results, a decision on whether the individual will be allowed to continue to drive.

If you are concerned about your parents' ability to drive, you can request an independent assessment for one or both of them. Such assessments, which are provided by private companies for a fee, will help you determine your parents' safety while on the road. Contact the Saskatchewan Government Insurance, Medical Review Unit.

Saskatchewan Government Insurance, Medical Review Unit

Telephone: (Regina) 775-6176; 1-800-667-8015 ext. 6176
Website: www.sgi.sk.ca/sgi_internet; Email: mruinquires@sgi.sk.ca

Provides driver assessments to determine driving competence.

YUKON

GOVERNMENT

For a full list of programs and services offered by the federal government, please refer to FEDERAL GOVERNMENT in the Canada-wide listings.

Home care and long-term care services are accessed throughout the territory by calling the government departments listed below or 1-800-661-0408.

Extended Health Care Benefits for Seniors

Telephone: 867-667-5403

Range of health services for elderly people who are not covered by private insurance.

Home Care/Home Support Program

Telephone: 867-667-5774

This government office will refer callers to numerous home care services such as occupational and physical therapy, nursing, and social work. It also provides home care services such as personal care, support activities, health and safety, and bathing.

Seniors Information Centre

Telephone: 867-668-3383

Website: www.users.yknet.yk.ca/yukonseniors/sic.html;

Email: ycoa@yknet.yk.ca

Funded through Yukon Council on Aging, the centre provides information on federal, territorial, municipal, and other programs for seniors. Publishes *Information Please: A Handbook for Yukon Seniors and Elders*, a helpful guide to seniors' services.

GENERAL RESOURCES/SPECIAL NEEDS

Alzheimer Society of British Columbia

Telephone: 1-800-667-3742

Email: info@alzheimerbc.org

The Alzheimer Society provides educational and support programs to improve awareness and to assist families and individuals coping with the disease, as well as telephone support for families and caregivers throughout the province. Regional representatives, respite managers, and volunteers can be contacted by phone or at a regional resource centre. An information package with more local material and a comprehensive facilities list can be requested at no charge. The British Columbia branch provides services to Yukon residents.

Arthritis Society, BC & Yukon Division

Telephone: 604-714-5550 or 1-800-321-1433
Website: www.arthritis.ca/bc; Email: info@bc.arthritis.ca

A non-profit organization devoted to funding and promoting arthritis research, patient care, and public education. Check the website or call the toll-free number above to find the offices and services nearest you.

Canadian Cancer Society, BC & Yukon Division

Telephone: 604-872-4400 or 1-800-663-2524
Cancer Information Service: 1-888-939-3333
Website: www.bc.cancer.ca; General email: inquiries@bc.cancer.ca
For information about cancer: info@cis.cancer.ca

Each division office provides various kinds of support and advice; call to find out what is available.

Canadian Diabetes Association, BC & Yukon

Telephone: 604-732-1331 or 1-800-665-6526
Website: www.diabetes.ca; Email: infobc@diabetes.ca

A national, independent, self-financing organization that works to improve the quality of life of Canadians affected by diabetes by being the leading force in research, service, advocacy, and education A very helpful website provides information to patients and professionals; patient information is available in English and Chinese. Call the number above for the office nearest you.

Canadian Hard of Hearing Association, Yukon Chapter

Telephone: 1-800-263-8068; (TTY) 613-526-2692
Email: chhanational@chha.ca

The association provides information and brochures on improving communication skills and helping people deal with hearing loss.

Canadian Mental Health Association, Yukon Division

Telephone: 867-668-7144

Email: deliasmorgan@yahoo.com

Provides information and support on mental health issues.

Canadian National Institute for the Blind, BC-Yukon Division

Telephone: 250-563-1702

Website: www.cnib.ca/divisions/bc_yukon; Email: cheryl.nguyen@cnib.ca

The Canadian National Institute for the Blind offers numerous resources, including counselling and referral, orientation and mobility training, sight enhancement, and technical aids.

SeniorsCan Yukon Information

Website: www.crm.mb.ca/yk

The SeniorsCan Internet Program is a highly acclaimed guide for retirees and older adults to Canadian and global information and services. The website for Yukon information is still under development.

NURSING AND HOMEMAKING AGENCIES

For nursing and homemaking agencies in your area, please contact the Yukon Home Support Program at 867-667-5774.

HOME HEALTH CARE RETAILERS, HOME SAFETY AND ENVIRONMENT

A social/intake worker at the territorial home care program will be able to find you the home health care products you require. You'll also find products through the following private companies that operate in your region.

Alpine Health Supplies and Services

Telephone: 867-393-4967

Email: alpinehealth@knet.yk.ca

Provides a full line of medical supplies, ranging from wheelchairs to commodes, and all items an elderly person in need of special aids may require.

Canada Mortgage and Housing Corporation, British Columbia and Yukon Division

Telephone: 867-633-7530

Website: www.cmhc.ca

See the Canada-wide listing under HOME HEALTH CARE RETAILERS, HOME SAFETY, AND ENVIRONMENT for services offered. Call the above number or visit the website to find the office nearest you.

FINANCIAL PLANNING/LEGAL

Office of the Public Administrator

Telephone: 867-667-5366 or 1-800-661-0408 ext. 5366

Email: publicadministrator@gov.yk.ca

This office is responsible for protecting the financial rights of cognitively challenged people. It helps individuals make decisions on personal care and medical treatment and advises family members on guardianship and on how to obtain the legal authority to make decisions on behalf of loved ones.

DRIVING CAPABILITY ASSESSMENT

In each province and territory, the Ministry of Transportation makes the official decision on when a person must stop driving. Your family physician is legally required to report any case in which someone's driving ability may be impaired due to the progression of age or any resulting condition. The physician must file his or her report with a medical review board, which may, based on research and interviews with key health care professionals, request a driving assessment to determine driving competence. Based on test results, a decision will be made on whether the individual will be allowed to continue to drive.

If you are concerned about your parents' ability to drive, you can request an independent assessment for one or both of them. Such assessments, which are provided by private companies for a fee, will help you determine your loved one's safety while on the road. For a private assessment, please see DriveAble under the heading DRIVING CAPABILITY ASSESSMENT for British Columbia.

Yukon Community and Transportation Services, Motor Vehicles and Driver Licences

Telephone: (Whitehorse) 867-667-5315 or 1-800-661-0408 ext. 5315

This department provides driver assessments to determine driving competence. Call to find the office nearest you.